Hives of Sickness

A Publication of the Museum of the City of New York
Robert R. Macdonald, Director

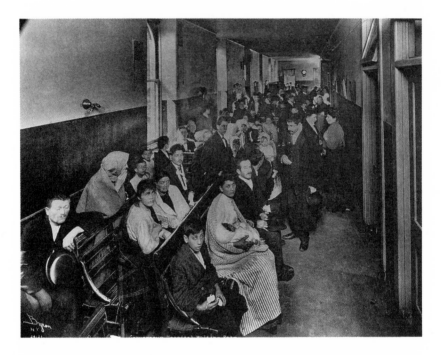

Gouverneur Hospital waiting room, 1906. The Byron Collection, Museum of the City of New York.

Hives of Sickness

PUBLIC HEALTH AND EPIDEMICS IN NEW YORK CITY

Edited by David Rosner

Published for the Museum of the City of New York by
RUTGERS UNIVERSITY PRESS
New Brunswick, New Jersey

Library of Congress Cataloging-in-Publication Data

Hives of sickness : public health and epidemics in New York City /
    edited by David Rosner.
        p.   cm.
    "Published for the Museum of the City of New York."
    Includes bibliographical references and index.
    ISBN 0-8135-2158-0
    1. Public health—New York (N.Y.)—History.   2. Communicable
diseases—New York (N.Y.)   I. Rosner, David, 1947–   . II. Museum
of the City of New York.
    [DNLM: 1. Urticaria—epidemiology—New York City.   2. Delivery of
Health Care—trends—New York City.   WR 170 H676 1995]
RA448.N5H54   1995
614.4'9747'1—dc20
DNLM/DLC
for Library of Congress   94-29784
                                                                                   CIP

British Cataloging-in-Publication information available

Contents

Robert R. Macdonald, Foreword   vii

David Rosner, Introduction: "Hives of Sickness and Vice"   1

PART I
Breeding Grounds for Disease   23

Gretchen A. Condran, Changing Patterns of Epidemic Disease in
New York City   27

Elizabeth Blackmar, Accountability for Public Health: Regulating the
Housing Market in Nineteenth-Century New York City   42

Alan M. Kraut, Plagues and Prejudice: Nativism's Construction of Disease
in Nineteenth- and Twentieth-Century New York City   65

PART II
When Epidemic Strikes   91

Judith Walzer Leavitt, "Be Safe. Be Sure.": New York City's Experience
with Epidemic Smallpox   95

Naomi Rogers, A Disease of Cleanliness: Polio in New York City,
1900–1990   115

Ronald Bayer, The Dependent Center: The First Decade of the AIDS
Epidemic in New York City   131

PART III
The City Responds   151

Elizabeth Fee and Evelynn M. Hammonds, Science, Politics, and the Art of
Persuasion: Promoting the New Scientific Medicine in New York City   155

Daniel M. Fox, The Politics of Public Health in New York City: Contrasting
Styles Since 1920   197

Notes on Contributors   211

Index   213

Foreword

Of all of the elements that embrace human experience, none has had a greater impact on the history of individuals and communities than health. The role of disease or, more accurately, the absence of physical and mental well-being, is so central to the understanding of the past and present that it is possible to view what has gone before from the perspective of those epidemics that have struck and that continue to plague societies throughout the world. The individual and collective reactions to these public health crises as well as the scientific responses to widespread sickness are mirrors to the cultural, religious, economic, political, and social histories of cities and nations.

Because the understanding of those histories is vital for a lucid comprehension of the present, the Museum of the City of New York, New York City's history museum, has developed this publication that places contemporary public health issues in historical context. *Hives of Sickness: Public Health and Epidemics in New York City* is the second in a series of projects organized by the museum that place subjects of concern to contemporary New York in historical context. The first of these projects studied the history of the homeless in New York through a scholarly symposium, exhibition, and book. In the future the museum plans to address such topics as the history of the New York Police Department, the idea of New York as the "melting pot," and how the city has planned its physical future.

This volume is the fruit of many dedicated professionals. David Rosner, the capable editor of this anthology, and the scholars who have participated in this work are owed a debt of gratitude by all those who care about New York City and its future.

This series of essays was made possible by a generous grant from the Josiah Macy, Jr., Foundation, Inc. I want to thank the foundation and its president, Dr. Thomas H. Meikle, Jr., for their confidence in the museum as well as their patience and advice in bringing the work to completion. It is the hope of all those associated with this project that by placing current public health emergencies in historical context we can address those issues with a wisdom gained through historical knowledge. History alone will not provide solutions, but without historical perspective, solutions are not possible.

Robert R. Macdonald
Director, Museum of the City of New York

Hives of Sickness

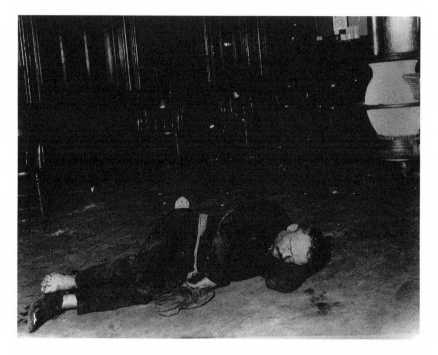

Police Station, Lodging House. Typhus victim. Undated photograph, c. 1890s.
The Jacob Riis Collection, Museum of the City of New York.

Introduction:
"Hives of Sickness and Vice"

Memory plays an immense trick on most of us who write about the history of New York. We often depend on memoirs that shroud the city's past in a glorious aura that contrasts dramatically with our view of today's city. In the writings of politicians, authors, and even historians, the city of past generations seems marvelously exciting, exhilarating, organized, and wholesome. In contrast, today's city seems overwhelmingly burdened with signs and symptoms of decay and dissolution. In the early 1970s, Otto Bettmann, who collected and catalogued thousands of photographs of nineteenth-century New York, characterized this process as the creation of a "benevolent haze" that leaves "us with the image of an ebullient, carefree America."[1]

This process of selective memory applies to writings about every period in the city's past. In the 1920s, writers remembered the decade of the "gay" nineties, much of which was spent in deep economic depression. Similarly, the 1920s were later remembered nostalgically, as were the 1940s and 1950s. A recent book on racial politics in New York speaks of the "breakdown" of the city in the 1960s and beyond, implying that the largely segregated decades before were benign and perhaps more socially cohesive and coherent.[2] Today, even the strife-filled 1960s are nostalgically recalled: "The New York days! . . . They seem far away now. . . . The stunning cosmo of the city at a time when everyone seemed to know everyone else . . . , its magic and majesty . . . , its teeming adventure . . . , the hard work and the gratification."[3] Even historical symbols of poverty and dislocation—such as life on the Lower East Side or arrival at Ellis Island at the turn of the century—now evoke sentimental remembrances.

Certainly, there are aspects of all these periods that should be recalled and even celebrated. But, as the history of disease in the city all too clearly illustrates, it is dangerous to lament the passing of supposedly golden eras and to characterize the present as a period of decline and disintegration. When we somberly reflect on the past, historians and laypeople alike know that "the world [of the late-nineteenth-century city] was in no way spared the problems we consider horrendously our own" whether they be homelessness, poverty, crime, or, most poignantly, disease.[4] Similarly, when we put aside our current and very specific fears of urban violence, homelessness, poverty, tuberculosis, or AIDS, we can see sides of the modern city that reflect its continuing vibrancy and even hope.

THE NINETEENTH-CENTURY URBAN ENVIRONMENT

This process of historical reconstruction is sometimes part of a broader political agenda that can focus attention on newcomers to the city as a cause, rather than the victims, of disruptions in the life of the community. This use was particularly important in the nineteenth century, when New York City underwent profound change as millions of people came from rural America and Europe and the city's environment and economy were transformed. Despite well-documented racial strife, class antagonisms, poverty, and the exploitation of women, antebellum New York can all too easily appear to be a time and place of relative cohesiveness and salubrity, especially when compared to the apparent disorder and poverty of the teeming industrial city of the late nineteenth century. The city's demographic and physical transformation was hard to miss as an English-speaking, largely Protestant community became, by the 1880s, home to thousands of Catholic and Jewish immigrants and poor. New York City, only decades before a regional commercial hub, emerged as the nation's foremost center of trade, industry, finance, and communication. Along with these changes went a profound reorganization in work, neighborhood, housing, family, and transportation. Homes, work sites, and offices, once clustered around the ports and commercial sites of lower Manhattan and Brooklyn's shoreline, spread to outlying areas of Long Island and Westchester.[5]

The Disease Environment

For many New Yorkers in the middle and late decades of the nineteenth century, those whose memories of the city stretched back a few decades, recent change augured both possibility and problems. On the one hand, New York was obviously emerging as the nation's preeminent center of commerce, culture, and wealth. The city's opera house, museums, plays, amusement parks, and music halls all indicated its cultural dynamism.[6] On the other hand, the city's poverty, illness, crowding, and "foreignness" appeared frightening. To older, largely Protestant New Yorkers, it was difficult to deny the connection between "plagues and people." Nor was it possible to avoid incorporating nativist beliefs into programs aimed at controlling disease. Smallpox, cholera, typhoid, yellow fever, and a host of intestinal diseases in the young and old alike accompanied the recognition of poverty, population increase, and immigration.

The fears of an elite class of antebellum New Yorkers who bemoaned the passing of a "golden age" in the city's history were in large measure nostalgic and highly selective. High death rates and pestilence had long affected rich and poor communities alike and long marked "with shame the great City of New York."[7] Yet patterns of disease in recent decades appeared to contemporaries to confirm the community's decay. By mid-century, New York had among the worst health statistics in the nation. Vital statistics gathered by the city showed that while one out of every forty-four people died in 1863 in Boston and one of forty-four in Philadelphia, New York's rate was one in thirty-six. Even when compared with European centers such as London and Liverpool, New York fared badly. In London and Liverpool, death rates had hovered around one in forty-five since the introduction of modern sanitary practices. Despite the fact that endemic conditions such as tuberculosis and diarrheal diseases among children were clearly much more important contributors to mortality in the city than were epidemic diseases, the appearance of scourges such as cholera had a very real significance as symbols of the apparent rapidity with which the city was being transformed. Mortality data were collected and presented in a way that highlighted the city's apparent decline.[8]

New York did not first turn its attention to the "conditions of the poor" in mid-century, but never before had there been such a generalized sense that poor health was becoming a permanent aspect of the city's life. Investigations of the conditions of the poor had been conducted by such civic leaders as John Griscom as early as the 1840s, but underlying the early studies was the belief that disease, poor housing, and "immoral" conditions were largely isolated to certain "susceptible" or unworthy individuals and communities. In 1859, reformers organized the New York Sanitary Association in order to agitate on behalf of a new permanent administrative body capable of responding to the city's environmental crisis. Shortly thereafter, during the Civil War, the Sanitary Association joined with the newly formed New York Citizens' Association. In 1864, the Citizens' Association organized a Special Council of Hygiene and Public Health, whose first agenda item was to document the horrifying changes that had overtaken the city in the previous few decades. The association organized a district-by-district, block-to-block inspection of living conditions in Manhattan.[9]

Documenting Disease and Death

In 1865, the Association of New York issued its final report, *Sanitary Condition of the City*. Dedicated to the benefit of "all classes in the city," the report provided more than three hundred pages of detailed description of the city's physical, social, and moral character. Coming at the end of a bloody war that had cleaved not only the nation but the communities of the city as well, the report reflected both the hopes and fears of the merchant leaders who had commissioned it. Widely distributed in a variety of forms—a book, booklets, and pamphlets—the report was used to pressure the city and the state to organize a permanent Metropolitan Board of Health the following year. Hamilton Fish, John Jacob Astor, Jr., Robert Roosevelt, August Belmont, and other members of elite merchant society had hoped that the city could embark on a reform effort that could lift it from the depths of disorder and disease. Advocating a permanent health department, they worried that only a permanent organization with police powers could possibly control the social forces of disorder fostered by the changing character of both the population and the commercial economy.

In order to accomplish the enormous task of first documenting the reasons for the high disease and death rates in the city and then developing a plan for public and private action, the council called upon New York's leading physicians to participate in a fact-gathering expedition. Valentine Mott, the "father of vascular surgery," Willard Parker, the first American to remove an appendix successfully, John Griscom, the author of the famous 1845 study of the *Sanitary Conditions of [New York's] Laboring Population,* Stephen Smith, soon to head New York's new Metropolitan Board of Health and found the American Public Health Association, and other prominent physicians and civic leaders agreed to participate in a systematic inspection of the city's various sanitary inspection districts. Beginning with the observation that "pestilential diseases" laid bare "the impotence of the existing sanitary system," the physicians noted that outbreaks of disease paralyzed the commercial and political life of the community: "The people are panic-stricken [and] the interests of commerce suffer by the insensible and certain *loss of millions.*" In a city of fewer than one million people, fully seven thousand to ten thousand lives could be saved, it was estimated, if proper sanitary practices could be developed.[10] It was clear that "the relation of the health and vigorous life of a people to the State, or to commercial prosperity, requires no discussion." Disease was a commodity in the developing commercial capital that could be measured in dollars and cents. An organized response to the high disease rates was a political and social necessity.

The recent war had illustrated only too clearly that living conditions directly affected well-being and health. "Reformatory efforts, whether social or political or exclusively moral and religious," were of "paramount necessity," as illustrated by the 1863 draft riots that had so traumatized the city. "The mobs that held fearful sway in our city during the memorable out-break of violence in the month of July, 1863, were gathered in the overcrowded and neglected quarters of the city," the committee report reminded readers. "The high brick blocks and closely-packed houses where the mobs originated seemed to be literally *hives of sickness and vice.*" The report went on to point out sardonically,

> It was wonderful to see, and difficult to believe, that so much misery, disease, and wretchedness can be huddled together and hidden by high walls, unvisited and unthought of, so near our own abodes. Lewd but pale and sickly young women, scarcely decent in their ragged attire, were impudent and scattered everywhere in the

crowd. But what numbers are made hideous by self-neglect and infirmity! . . . To walk the streets as we walked them, in those hours of conflagration and riot, was like witnessing the day of judgement, with every wicked thing revealed, every sin and sorrow blazingly glared upon, every hidden abomination laid before hell's expectant fire. . . .

The elements of popular discord are gathered in those wretchedly-constructed tenant-houses, where poverty, disease, and crime find an abode. Here disease in its most loathsome form propagates itself. Unholy passions rule in the domestic circle. Everything, within and without, tends to physical and moral degradation.[11]

The observation that housing, politics, morals, and health were all inter-twined underscored the committee's perception of what needed to be done in the coming years. Of first importance was the need to document and quantify the degree of suffering, the inadequacy of services and horrors of urban life. Hence, members of the committee set out to expose "themselves to repulsive and nauseous scenes in the abodes of misery and want, and to the infectious localities and homes of disease and death, in order to be able to give an exact and complete survey of the sufferings, perils, and sanitary wants."[12] With a voyeur's acuity, an elite's sense of authority, and the moral righteousness of missionaries, the report was a remarkable document that detailed the physical and social life of mid-nineteenth-century New York.

The Setting

New York was, in 1865, still geographically identical with Manhattan Island, located between the Hudson and East rivers and bounded on the north by Westchester, the east by Brooklyn and Long Island, and on the west by New Jersey. The island, far from being a level, neatly laid out grid of rectangular blocks, was marked by hills and gullies, streams, marshlands, and meadows. Much of the shoreline had been filled in over the preceding decades, yet areas along the rivers still had large pockets of swamp and wetlands. The densely populated area between Houston Street and Fourteenth Street and as far west as Tompkins Square was an uneven marshland, while just to the north along the water's edge lay land filled with the rubble, granite, and earth excavated from the center of the island. The sparsely populated sections of the city north from Central Park were all the more uneven, with cliffs and valleys, streams and meadows.

The report can be used as a walking guide through a city that appeared to the committee to be on the verge of anarchy and collapse. In descriptions of the various neighborhoods, we find a wealth of information about the infra-structure of a city that was doubling in population nearly every decade. The location of sewers, natural springs, ponds, and rock formations are detailed. We also can discern the environmental balance that had been disrupted by the city's rapid economic and demographic development. Just north of City Hall, for example, in the area now occupied by the Tombs and other city and federal buildings, lay an area that had been, in the early nineteenth century, a pure-water pond known as the Collect. In 1800, it was the "largest pond on Manhattan Island," surrounded by groves, fields, and a "high hill rising abruptly from its sides." Its waters had been of "great depth and of unusual purity," providing nearly ten thousand New Yorkers with fresh spring water.[13]

Yet, beginning in the early 1800s, the Collect was filled in as its value for tenement housing became apparent to the emerging landlord class. Quickly, the Collect became a dumping ground for dead animals and offal, giving the area "an insufferable stench." Then a canal was dug from the Collect along Canal Street to the Hudson, and the area was graded to allow for commercial traffic through its crowded streets. By the end of the Civil War, the area was covered with tenements "containing 4 to 8 families in as many rooms." The lodging houses of the area had "as many as thirty persons . . . packed into one small room," promoting, as in the case of one such house on Baxter Street, large and virulent outbreaks of fever.[14]

The description of the area provided the Sanitary Commission with a vivid understanding of how the intimate relationship between social and economic forces created a slum and ill health throughout the district. The commercial avenues of the area were paved with cobblestones, which, in turn, provided deep cracks in which refuse collected and rotted. The streets were "very filthy," with accumulations of manure from the horses that traversed the area, dead dogs, cats, and rats; and household and vegetable refuse that in winter accumulated to depths of three feet or more. "Garbage boxes," rarely emptied, overflowed with offal, animal carcasses, and household waste. "Pools" of stagnant water collected in the carcasses of dead animals and over sewer drains that were generally clogged. "Filth of every kind [was] thrown into the streets, covering their surface, filling the gutters, obstructing the sewer culverts, and sending forth perennial emanations which must generate pestiferous diseases," reported William Thoms, the sanitary inspector for the district. "Drainage is generally imperfect, the courtyards being . . . below the level of the streets," and "everything is thrown into the street and gutters at all times of the day."[15] Poorly designed sewers had been installed throughout the region, but most of the population depended upon the outdoor "water closets" and privies in the courtyards of the tenement buildings, close to wells used for drinking.

The few amenities provided were generally inadequate, often becoming public health hazards themselves. The water closets were generally "covered and surrounded with filth, so as not to be approachable." Others were "merely trenches sunken one or two feet in the ground, the fluids of which [were] in some instances allowed to run into the courts, stones and boards . . . provided to keep the feet out of filth." Half the houses in the district had no sewers connected to them, making the stench that arose during the summer "absolutely unbearable and perilous."[16] Twenty-nine brothels, 43 stables, and 406 "dram shops" added to the generalized decay of a district that seventy-five years before had boasted the purest water in the city.

Most obvious to the various inspectors who wrote the district reports was the stench that characterized the city's poor sections. In district after district, the inspectors detailed the smell of "sewer gas" that escaped the inadequate sewerage system, the polluted water supply, the filthy streets, the overflowing garbage, the collapsing tenement houses and other airless, overcrowded fire-traps. Inspector after inspector worried that the "miasmas" created by rotting foods and filth threatened the neighborhood, and the larger city as well. They feared that the worthy and the unworthy, the young and the old, the rich and the poor all were susceptible to the fevers and plagues that were carried through the air. "Familiar with the haunts of fever and other pestilential diseases, the Sanitary Inspectors have fearlessly penetrated the dismal and unwholesome quarters where infectious poisons and deadly maladies menace inhabitants and visitants, and from whence emanate the most dreaded diseases that find their way to the more favored districts of the city."[17] In New York, "disease, debasement, and pauperism . . . are found closely allied" and "seriously endanger the sanitary safety of all other classes.[18]

The report accepted that the "fever-nests and small-pox fields that infest[ed] the city" were neither inevitable nor "natural." Rather, infectious disease was controllable through social reordering and administrative action. The report observed that "come what events there may be to affect the physical, social, political, or commercial interests of the city, let it be borne in mind that Sanitary Science and its preventive skill are of more value to our fellow beings and to this city than all the curative arts of medicine and surgery."[19] The report suggested a program of street cleaning, building sewers and pure-water supplies, garbage collection, and meat and milk inspection.

Death and Disease in the New Environment

Despite the relative abundance of land across the Hudson River in New Jersey, across the East River on Long Island, and to the north in Westchester or what we now know as the Bronx, the pattern of building, economic development, and land use had created in New York some of the world's worst crowding and most depressing health statistics. By the middle years of the century, epidemics of typhus, yellow fever, cholera, and other diseases swept through the tenements and slums of the city with fearsome impact. Despite the fact that epidemics were relatively minor contributors to overall death rates, the highly visible and often dramatic experience of seeing people literally dying in the streets had an enormous impact, affecting where and how the city developed. In the late eighteenth century, yellow fever had caused elite New Yorkers to flee north from New York to the then-salubrious and relatively distant suburb of Greenwich Village. In later years, as the city's population grew and the concentration of people in crowded downtown areas increased, the creation of newer communities in the upper reaches of the island promised safety and health in return for inconvenience. Some began long, almost impossible commutes from Brooklyn by ferry and from Bloomingdale and distant Harlem by wagon, horse and carriage, and, late in the century, electric trolley, to the wharves, stores, and financial and commercial centers downtown.

In part, the extraordinary crowding that characterized the city in the midnineteenth century was produced by its unique economy and topography. Built as a port and located on an island without bridges, tunnels, efficient transportation, or communication, the city's population originally concentrated in the relatively narrow band of land between the two rivers. Yet, more important, economic and topographic forces played a role in creating midnineteenth-century New York's wretched living conditions. The commercial city had created a skewed market for land and housing; this provided landlords and absentee owners with enormous profits and denied the workers and their families wholesome living quarters. Early-eighteenth-century housing patterns in which artisans and working people lived and worked in the same dwelling were replaced by land-use patterns that separated work from home, wealthy from poor, immigrant from native, owner from occupant. The market for housing, as Elizabeth Blackmar details, created "unnatural" social relationships and market-driven scarcities of housing and land, which, in turn, created the preconditions for the disastrous health experience that the committee confronted as market values replaced human values in the city's legal and social environment.[20] In response to this transformation of the housing market and physical environment, and accompanying social disruption, the city created a permanent institution, a department of public health, as a part of its attempt to regulate conditions that caused disease. Housing inspectors, meat and milk inspection, garbage collection and street cleaning, water distribution, and sewerage services would all be organized through a health department that sought to control the environment. Soon, the newly organized Department of Public Health would become a model for other cities throughout the nation, employing what were considered the latest "scientific" advances in bacteriology.

This book traces aspects of the public health crises that the council outlined in its mammoth document, as well as the responses to those crises. It also seeks to look at the various institutions, individuals, and diseases that have shaped our understanding of infectious disease. Although the report played a crucial role in the political drama surrounding the creation of New York's public health department, conditions for many New Yorkers continued to be marginal at best. In the years following its creation, the Health Department would focus on cleaning the streets, regulating sewerage and waste disposal, and mandating tenement reforms such as the development of indoor privies and direct connections to sewer systems. It would also seek to become a leader in the evolving movement to develop a scientific base to public health practice. By the turn of the twentieth century, New York would emerge as preeminent in the field. Older sanitarians' notions of the cause of disease as residing in filth and immorality would slowly be supplemented with newer, ostensibly scientific views that disease was caused by specific pathogens, bacteria, associated with specific diseases. The new thinking was that attacking the means by which particular pathogens spread, rather than engaging in programs of fumigation or street cleanups, would be more economically efficient and more effective in stopping the spread of disease. The isolation of diseased individuals, the vaccination of potential victims of infection, and laboratory analysis of milk supplies slowly gained a place alongside the more traditional sanitarian focus of the public health department.[21] Simultaneously, these older traditional public health programs were moved to new departments of sanitation and charity.

Before the 1880s, public health workers had a different conception of health than did clinicians. While physicians saw sick patients and sought to identify the cause of disease and treat its symptoms, public health workers addressed the problem of environmental control, developing a perspective that emphasized personal and public hygiene. Sanitation, the inspection of meats, sewage, housing, immigration control, and the provision of clean water and air were critical to the mandate of the public health professional.

Tuberculosis, the Germ Theory, and Public Health Practice

The sanitarians who led reform efforts generally saw themselves as more than technical experts or trained professionals. Some had come from elite merchant families, and others had been trained in the ministry. They defined their mission as much in moral as in secular terms and believed that illness, filth, and disorder were intrinsically related. Individual transgression and social decay were equally causative of poor health. In the period before widespread acceptance of the notion that there was a specific pathogen for a particular disease entity, public health, medical practitioners, and laypeople alike understood disease in highly personal and idiosyncratic terms. Much of public health practice as well as medical therapeutics rested on the belief that disease was a reflection of individuals' special social, personal, hereditary, and economic circumstances. As Charles Rosenberg has written, "The body was seen, metaphorically, as a system of dynamic interactions with its environment. Health or disease resulted from a cumulative interaction between constitutional endowment and environmental circumstance."[22] It was the special relationship between an individual and a complex, highly particularized environment that was at the root of illness. The practitioner's therapeutic skill was measured by his or her ability to weigh, evaluate, and differentiate the patient from others who might have similar symptoms. While the medical practitioner addressed those peculiarities of the individual that might predispose him or her to disease, public health practitioners defined their mission in terms of the broader environment within which populations lived. Rather than being technicians who administered a universal cure or standardized medical regimen for a set of complaints, medical practitioners for much of the century saw themselves as responsible for adjusting dosages, altering prescriptions, and changing regimens as conditions demanded. Public health practice looked into the peculiar environmental conditions of housing, nutrition, or employment but also saw solutions arising from much broader environmental manipulations such as street sweeping or providing pure water supplies to the larger community.

The prevention, diagnosis, and treatment of tuberculosis, "the great white plague," commonly called consumption and phthisis (a descriptive term derived from the Greek, meaning "to waste away"), developed within this general milieu. Despite the attention paid to epidemics of smallpox, cholera, or typhoid, tuberculosis was the single most important disease in nineteenth-century New York. For the previous two centuries, this condition had been the greatest cause of death in Europe and America. The symptoms of wasting away, coughing, spitting, and weakening appeared in victims from various classes and social strata.[23] The disease took on different meanings for different classes and groups in the changing urban and industrial societies of western Europe and the United States, however. Physicians "faced with a confusing array of signs and symptoms, bearing no obvious relation to one another," saw these signs as "the expression of different maladies." For middle-class sufferers the disease was often presented in an almost romantic light. The translucent flush of Victorian ladies suffering from this disease became a standard image in the nineteenth-century novel. For the working class, however, the disease had a much more threatening aspect: workers and their families huddled together in the slum dwellings of large cities such as London, Paris, and New York.[24]

The apparent idiosyncracy of the symptoms that marked phthisis among different individuals and social classes during most of the first half of the nineteenth century reinforced standard ideas regarding the nature, course, and treatment of disease. Phthisis could be linked to the ongoing, long-term moral and social environment that predisposed a victim to a disease process. Medical practitioners and the public as well shared a common set of assumptions about the cause and treatment of the disease. Phthisis could be rooted in personal behavior such as drinking, social position, poor living quarters, the malaise of an urban lifestyle, and indoor, unhealthful work. "Treatment was to be sensitively gauged not to a disease entity but to such distinctive features of the patient as age, gender, ethnicity, socioeconomic position, and moral status, and to attributes of place like climate, topography and population density."[25] A practitioner needed a complete knowledge of the life history of the patient in order to make an accurate diagnosis and plan of treatment. Public health practitioners had to understand the environmental conditions that allowed for the disease's spread.

Public health practitioners such as Hermann Biggs in New York City, Charles Chapin in Rhode Island, and others had documented the importance of a variety of sources for phthisis. Among them were conditions in the home and crowding, impure air, and dust in the workplace. In New York City in 1879, Roger Tracy, the registrar of vital statistics, noted the symptoms of disease among workers in the metal trades. "The disease comes on very gradually . . . and its duration may be extended over four or five years." He described that the disease "begins with the cough of irritation, dry and hacking at first, with very scanty expectoration, whitish and stringy in character. . . . The expectoration gradually increases in amount and becomes reddish, and soon after this tinge appears there may be haemoptysis."[26]

Consumption, or phthisis, had a varied set of symptoms. It could be of an acute nature and "prove fatal in a few weeks." Or it might start with acute symptoms and evolve into a chronic condition. Its symptoms might appear slowly, gradually getting worse over many years. It could affect lungs, bones, the brain, and other organs of the body. Pulmonary consumption was of primary importance, but the variety of symptoms, prognoses, and sites gave medical researchers a basis for developing a complex and all-encompassing nosology.

In the years following Pasteur's work on rabies and the bacterial origins of yeast, the medical community began to change its views regarding the multiple sources of illness. Increasingly, laboratory science began to hold out the possibility that disease could be explained rationally through the discovery of specific microorganisms. For the practitioner, this meant that the detailed life history was no longer as essential for understanding the diagnosis of disease. Although medical practitioners continued to speak of the significance of the "history" in diagnosing patient's illnesses, the concept of a medical history changed.

In the years following Koch's discovery of the tuberculosis bacillus, medical history became a listing of physiological and hereditary factors that might explain the symptom. "In attempting to arrive at a correct solution of the problem," noted one physician explaining the method of diagnosing tuberculosis in 1904, "the greatest care should always be exercised to ascertain and carefully [list] all the facts that can be learned concerning the patient's past history and mode of life." In the middle years of the nineteenth century this might have meant exploring personal behavior, work history, and living conditions, but by now it simply meant examining "the probable duration of the disease, the occurrence of a foregoing haemoptysis, a history of an attack of typhoid pneumonia, pleurisy, or protracted influenza, and, to a certain extent the individual's appearance."[27] The impact of this changing medical culture was critical in the study of phthisis.[28] The disease came to be understood as tuberculosis, caused by a specific organism and spread like other infectious diseases. "Medical science claims that the presence of the tubercle bacillus in the lungs is the fundamental cause of phthisis, or consumption," trumpeted a New Yorker writing to *Scientific American* in 1904.[29]

For the public health and medical fields, the trick was to reconcile the myriad of symptoms with the new "scientific" germ model. After all, the discovery of the bacillus held out the possibility that an effective vaccine could be developed to protect humanity from this age-old scourge. "We are now anxiously waiting the development of Dr. Koch's cure for consumption," said one professor of pathology at the University of Michigan in 1890.[30]

With the revolution in bacteriology that followed the discoveries of Pasteur, Lister, and Koch in the middle decades of the nineteenth century, a new faith in laboratory science had emerged not only among physicians but also among public health workers. "Bacteriology thus became an ideological marker, sharply differentiating the 'old' public health, the province of untrained amateurs, from the 'new' public health, which belonged to scientifically trained professionals," points out Elizabeth Fee.[31] Despite the different professional mandates of public health workers and physicians, members of both professions who identified themselves with the science of medicine and public health began to share a common faith in the significance of the disease-specific germ entity in creating consumption. The implications for professional and public health understanding were that the modes of transmission of the bacteria had to be clearly identified if an effective campaign to eliminate the sources of the disease was to be mounted. Why were the poor so likely to be struck by disease? Because the hot, crowded dwellings in which they lived allowed the germ to propagate and to spread among a population weakened by inadequate nutrition and horrid living conditions. Why did children appear to be a high-risk group? Because tainted milk from tubercular cows poisoned children. How did individuals outside any particular risk group come down with the disease? Because they had a hereditary predisposition that left them vulnerable to infection. Why did workers have a higher rate of tuberculosis than farmers? Because close quarters combined with long hours and inadequate diet to leave them susceptible to phthisis.

For the new public health, it was the specificity of the bacterial agent that was important. The older generation's emphasis on cleaning up the general environment seemed misdirected and inefficient. One of the advocates of the new public health summed up the revolution in ideology that overtook the field in the 1880s: "Before 1880 we knew nothing; after 1890 we knew it all; it was a glorious ten years."[32] A new model was gaining greater acceptance: a bacillus made people sick and phthisis was caused by germs that propagated in stagnant air.[33] The slums of large cities came to be seen as "breeding grounds" that were "seeded" with tuberculosis bacilli waiting to infect the susceptible victim. Tuberculosis came to be viewed as a disease that could be transmitted to susceptible individuals by means of air impregnated with bacteria from dried sputum, breathing, and other sources. Dusting furniture could throw into the air the "dried sputum" of tuberculars. Crowded public spaces or unclean home conditions with moist, warm, and stagnant air were seen as the most likely conduits for the disease.[34]

The prospect of bacteriological explanations held promise not only that specific cures and preventive vaccines could be developed but also that focusing on specific disease-prevention programs could result in more efficient uses of public health resources. "A careless or ignorant expectorating consumptive can eliminate and distribute seven billions of bacilli in twenty-four hours," warned S. A. Knopf in the journal *Charities* in 1901.[35] Hence, by encouraging the tuberculous to carry and use flasks to dispose of their spittle so that "it cannot dry and be blown about to be inhaled by others," journals declared that responsible tuberculars could stem the disease. Public health policies that focused on the sources of specific infection reather than on the general sanitary conditions of the broader city had numerous attractions. Among them was the prospect of efficiently stemming infection without disrupting existing social relationships between tenant and landlord, employer and worker, political leaders and voters. Health and wealth could both be attained.[36]

The relative simplicity, usefulness, and cohesiveness of the germ theory of disease was incorporated into older sanitarian notions regarding the relationship between cleanliness, godliness, and health. The need for a synthesis was pressed on public health leaders by a diverse group of Progressive Era reformers who were concerned with the plight of the urban poor in the newly emerging industrial capitalism of the city and country. They continually pressed the point that disease could not be divorced from the terrible conditions of life and work and that health and social problems had to be addressed together. Charity and settlement house workers, for example, documented that nearly one out of every four dwellings in New York City in 1890 experienced a death from phthisis. In the poorer neighborhoods, it was clear, the toll was much higher, leaving these communities devastated by the disease.[37] For these reformers, phthisis was a disease of poverty as much as it was one of germs. One of the leading social welfare reformers of the time, Graham Taylor, declared that tuberculosis was a "disease of the working classes" and that "everything which makes the life of the workingman harder, everything which is attendant upon poverty, makes for the increase of this disease."[38] "Housing, playgrounds, diet, income, . . . physical education, . . . immigration" and even dental hygiene "appear to be very diverse if not incongruous topics, [but when] grouped about the central idea of promoting immunity their interdependence becomes obvious."[39]

Especially clear was the connection between work and tuberculosis.[40] "Where there is dirt and grime and dust, long hours, foul air and bad pay, the community pays for what it calls cheap prices by a little money and many lives sacrificed to greed, ignorance and indifference," pointed out one labor representative in 1906.[41] Graham Taylor saw four "characteristics of employment" that put workers at risk: "insanitary conditions," "low rate of wages," "fatigue," and "long and irregular hours." Under the heading of insanitary conditions, Taylor identified two major subcategories: "hygienic surroundings which are not inherent in the trade itself and those conditions which are to a certain extent necessitated by the character of the trade."[42]

TWENTIETH-CENTURY PUBLIC HEALTH

A half-century after the Citizens' Association report, the city's public health officials were continuing to adjust and incorporate new ideas into older patterns of practice. Further, they were incorporating the germ theory into older notions regarding the relationship of the changing urban environment and the health of its people. In large measure because of the efforts of the organizers of the 1865 report, the city now had in place a permanent department of health with responsibility for controlling some of the city's worst environmental problems. Garbage collection, meat and milk inspections, pure water, and sewerage systems had been installed throughout the city. Dead animals were now regularly picked up off the streets, and fire safety codes augmented stricter enforcement of housing laws. Yet serious and pervasive problems persisted, and the types of diseases the city faced appeared to be changing. Neither smallpox, the classic epidemic disease of the eighteenth and nineteenth centuries, nor polio, a twentieth-century terror, would be completely controlled until after World War II.

New Public Health and Old Health Conditions

Despite decades of agitation and a rapidly evolving view of disease causation, the Department of Health still faced daunting environmental hazards. In 1912, it issued an annual report that, in language as dispassionate as any, detailed the continuing environmental problems that New Yorkers faced. The department picked up over 20,000 dead horses, mules, donkeys, and cattle from the city's streets during the year and recorded 343,000 complaints from citizens, inspectors, and officials about problems ranging from inadequate ventilation, and leaking cesspools and water closets to unlicensed manure dumps and animals kept without permits. The department also removed nearly half a million smaller animals such as pigs, hogs, calves, and sheep. Furthermore, its meat inspection unit removed 5,669,470 pounds of spoiled poultry, fish, offal, pork, and beef and carted 1,946 cubic yards of night soil from the backyards and privies of the city's tenements.[43]

The scope of activities had expanded enormously over the course of the previous half-century, and the department's budget now amounted to nearly four million dollars. Significantly, a "remarkable and continuous decrease in the death rate . . . accompanied the development . . . of public sanitation," the report began. "In 1866, the year in which the department was organized, the death rate of New York City was 36.31 per thousand." The rate continued to decline decade after decade, and had recently fallen to below 16 per thousand. The department was justifiably proud: over the course of just forty-five years, there was a decrease of over 50 percent.[44]

"Public Health Is Purchasable": New Health Issues Emerge

Somewhat startling, however, was the emergence of changing patterns of death in the city. The report's author wondered whether the nature of disease in the city was undergoing a perceptible shift. "An enormous reduction in mortality [had] taken place in all age groups below forty-five, while there has [been] an actual increase in the mortality at all ages over forty-five." The infectious diseases of the nineteenth century such as smallpox, typhoid fever, diphtheria, and pulmonary tuberculosis appeared to be claiming fewer and fewer of the city's children and young adults. Cancer, heart disease, and pneumonia were claiming larger and larger numbers of elderly, however. "Without exception," the report quizzically pointed out, "the diseases in which a reduction of mortality has been effected belong to the class of infectious diseases, while of those diseases in which there has been increase in the mortality only one, pneumonia, belongs to that group." To the public health officials writing the annual report, "these facts [were] doubly significant." On the one hand, they showed "in an unmistakable manner the success of public sanitary administration which has heretofore directed its efforts almost entirely against infectious diseases." On the other hand, they "point[ed] with equal clearness toward the field in which public hygiene must [focus] in the future, namely, the reduction of mortality from the diseases of middle and old age."[45] What new techniques could be employed to address these new challenges? Were the traditional tools of environmental cleanup or the newer techniques of vaccination and medical interventions adequate?

Unlike the moral undertone of the report of 1866, which had laid the groundwork for the creation of the department, the 1912 annual report used decidedly different language to describe the progress of the past five decades. The victory of sanitary science over the disease toll of poverty and commercial development pointed to some lessons that appeared self-evident in early-twentieth-century America: "Generally speaking, a study of the vital statistics of New York or any community can hardly fail to indicate the enormous advances achieved by sanitary science in the past fifty years. Since the full benefits of the methods and practice of sanitary science are available to any intelligent and well-organized community which will make the necessary expenditures, it may be truly said that within certain limits *public health is purchasable.*"[46]

The moral tone of the 1866 Citizens' Association report was replaced with new, professional, and technocratic approaches to controlling infectious diseases. Cleaning the streets, improving sewerage systems, providing pure water, and quarantining the sick became administrative and organizational feats that were accomplished without the moral and political fervor that had marked earlier reform efforts. For many in the city, infectious diseases became less of a threat, and New Yorkers undoubtedly benefited, as measured both by declining mortality and lowered costs, from the improved environments. Public health supplemented its original mission to prevent disease with a new mission to attack the specific sources of disease through the use of the laboratory, medical science, individual treatment, and the identification and sometimes isolation of individuals capable of spreading disease.[47]

The culmination of fifty years of political struggles to establish the department as an important arm of the city's administration had left it with a new mandate and a changing set of problems. No longer would public health be limited to environmental engineering and food inspection. In future years it would find itself coming into conflict with providers of medical care as disease prevention through inoculation and vaccination, prenatal and well-baby care, factory inspection, and occupational-disease prevention as well as treatment of communicable diseases such as syphilis and gonorrhea would force the field to venture into areas previously the preserve of physicians. Further, the emergence of chronic diseases and the apparent decline of infectious illness challenged the department to redefine its mission and elaborate a new purpose and role. By the 1970s, just before the reemergence of communicable diseases such as AIDS and tuberculosis as pressing health problems in the country, public health professionals would venture into a wide range of policy and administrative areas.

CHANGING NOTIONS OF DISEASE

The essays in this book are suggestive of a research agenda for the future. Together, they illustrate that the health problems we face as a city are largely of our own making and also are potentially under our own control. Our current fatalism notwithstanding, AIDS, tuberculosis, and diseases associated with poverty and homelessness are in a very real way social creations and therefore can be addressed through social decisions. In a recent essay on what he calls "framing" disease, Charles Rosenberg notes that "disease is at once a biological event, a generation-specific repertoire of verbal constructs reflecting medicine's intellectual and institutional history," and "a sanction for cultural values." Pointing out that disease is a "social phenomenon," he indicates that in large measure "disease does not exist until we have agreed that it does, by perceiving, naming, and responding to it."[48] Yet disease takes specific forms at different moments in history. Not only do we define different symptoms as pathological events, we also create the physical environments and social relationships that allow for the emergence of very real new problems. We create our environment, and hence we create the conditions within which diseases thrive. Whether cholera, silicosis, or yellow fever in the nineteenth century, or AIDS, cancer, heart disease, or tuberculosis today, the manner in which we address disease becomes emblematic of a specific society at a particular moment in history. Just as physicians, the elites, and the politicians in the middle nineteenth century presented cholera as a moral as well as medical stigma, so, too, do we use disease as metaphor. We need only recall that as recently as a decade ago newspapers, politicians, and public health professionals presented AIDS as a disease peculiar to Haitians and gay men to realize how deeply social values and specific historical circumstance shape our understanding of disease and how quickly our assumptions about the causes and victims of disease can change.

As we enter the second decade of the AIDS epidemic, certain statements that only a decade ago may have been provocative now seem self-evident. But epidemic disease has marked and shaped life in America's premier city for much of the nineteenth and twentieth centuries. For a few decades midway through this century most health analysts optimistically believed that infectious diseases were "conquered" or problems of the past. The reappearance of virulent strains of tuberculosis, the pandemic of AIDS, and the outbreaks of cholera in South and Central America raise anew the issue of whether such optimistic assessments were simply passing reflections of a generation's unbridled faith in the potential of curative medicine. This volume is intended to refocus our attention on the social responses to infectious diseases in their various forms and on our need to balance our belief in the possibilities of curing disease with the need to prevent them by improving the city's infrastructure, economy, and social and educational services, as well as its primary care and hospital system. Acute infectious diseases, such as cholera, yellow fever, typhoid, and typhus were as much part of the specific built environments that we as a culture created in the nineteenth century as are chronic disease such as heart disease and cancer, AIDS, and tuberculosis today. Specific diseases, and our responses to them, can be understood as concrete indicators of community and social relationships as well as discrete biological or socially negotiated entities. By focusing on New York City and on the demographic pressures as well as the economic and political responses to epidemic disease, this volume seeks to provide a window into the social world that helped "frame debates about society and social policy."[49]

Traditionally, we have defined epidemics as infectious disease that attack a population, causing high mortality and morbidity over a short period of time. Currently, we speak of a host of conditions that do not fit this classic model. Today we speak of drug use as epidemic, although the problem is clearly chronic in nature and is not related to a pathogen. Similarly, we describe cancer rates as being epidemic, although we generally think of cancer itself as a chronic, noninfectious disease. Alcohol use and car accidents, as well as AIDS, are all presented as epidemic despite the vast differences in prevalence, period of onset, symptoms, and treatments that separate them from nineteenth century epidemics of infection. As Charles Rosenberg details elsewhere, we use the word *epidemic* in a variety of ways that are neither linguistically or historically precise.[50]

In light of the ambiguity in the very meaning of *epidemic,* to edit a book that makes any pretense of comprehensiveness is either arrogant or meaningless. Hence, a brief caveat is in order for those readers who expect that this book will address the entire scope of epidemic disease or public health practice. Clearly, this volume is not meant as an encyclopedia of the history of epidemics in New York. Nor should one expect to find comprehensive essays on the scores of conditions that at different moments in history are considered epidemic. There are numerous books on different New York institutions that impacted on our disease experience, hundreds of reports on specific disease problems, and a handful of books on the history of particular epidemic diseases. Hospitals, dispensaries, social service agencies, city departments, immigrant histories, and the like all have something to say to the place of disease in New York. The Department of Health itself is the focus of John Duffy's massive two-volume work; Charles Rosenberg's *Cholera Years* is a book about just one disease during one century; and my own book on hospitals in the city is necessarily cursory, focusing on the short period of thirty years.[51]

It is hoped, however, that this volume will add to an ongoing discussion of the ways this community has created the environment for disease outbreaks, responded to the very diseases that plagued it, and built health into the agencies of government. Hence, the essays in the volume are grouped in three thematic sections. The first section, "Breeding Grounds for Disease," is composed of three essays about the disease environment of the nineteenth-century city and its relationship to broad changes in housing and population. The second section, "When Epidemic Strikes," addresses our experiences with three emblematic epidemic diseases—smallpox, polio, and AIDS—and seeks to look at different moments in the twentieth century during which changing social and scientific assumptions shaped our response. The final section of the book, "The City Responds," addresses the manner with which nineteenth- and twentieth-century New York organized and responded to epidemic disease. The first essay in this section outlines the activities of the city's Department of Health in the nineteenth and early twentieth centuries; the second essay outlines the transformation of the concept of public health in the twentieth century. New demands, coupled with changing ideas about the limits of public health, led to a subtle redefinition of the scope of the field and the responsibilities of public health officials. Together, these essays should be read as a contribution to the intellectual literature on the social and political history of the city. They should also serve to remind us that aspects of the current health crises in the city are not unique to this era and that, as in the past, a concerted effort to face up to modern epidemics can lead to meaningful and humanitarian responses.

Notes

1. Otto Bettmann, *The Good Old Days—They Were Terrible!* (New York: Random House, 1974), xi–xii. More recently, others have fondly and selectively remembered the "fresh spirit" of the New York of the 1920s and how "much of the New York" of that era "has been wildly changed." See William S. Hall, in *Christopher Morley's New York* (New York: Fordham University Press, 1988), xvi.

2. Jim Sleeper, *The Closest of Strangers: Liberalism and the Politics of Race in New York* (New York: W. W. Norton, 1990), 17.

3. Willie Morris, *New York Days* (New York: Little, Brown, 1993), 3.

4. Bettmann, *The Good Old Days*, xi–xii.

5. See, for example, Richard Wiebe, *The Search for Order, 1870–1920* (New York: Hill and Wang, 1966), which still ranks as one of the best overviews of the transformation of American life in the late nineteenth century.

6. See David Nasaw, *Going Out* (New York: Basic Books, 1993).

7. *Sanitary Condition of the City, Report of the Council of Hygiene and Public Health of the Citizens' Association of New York* (New York, 1865), xii.

8. *Sanitary Condition of the City*, xi. See also Charles Rosenberg, *The Cholera Years* (Chicago: University of Chicago Press, 1964), for what is still the best description of the shifting reaction of the city to this recurrent epidemic during the course of the nineteenth century.

9. John Duffy, *The Sanitarians: A History of American Public Health* (Urbana: University of Illinois Press, 1990), 118–119.

10. *Sanitary Condition of the City*, xii.

11. Ibid., xvi.

12. Ibid., xvii.

13. Ibid., 75.

14. Ibid., 77.

15. Ibid., 76.

16. Ibid., 80.

17. Ibid., xxxiv.

18. Ibid., cxliii.

19. Ibid., cxliii.

20. The significance of these changing economic and social relationships is detailed in Elizabeth Blackmar, *Manhattan for Rent, 1785–1850* (Ithaca: Cornell University Press, 1989), as well as in her essay in this volume.

21. Judith Leavitt, "'Typhoid Mary' Strikes Back, Bacteriological Theory and Practice in Early Twentieth Century Public Health," *ISIS* 83 (1992): 608–629.

22. Morris J. Vogel and Charles E. Rosenberg, *The Therapeutic Revolution: Essays in the Social History of American Medicine* (Philadelphia: University of Pennsylvania Press, 1979), 5.

23. René and Jean Dubos, *The White Plague: Tuberculosis, Man, and Society* (New Brunswick, N.J.: Rutgers University Press, 1987), 10. For an expanded discussion of

tuberculosis see David Rosner and Gerald Markowitz, *Deadly Dust: Silicosis and the Politics of Occupational Disease in Twentieth Century America* (Princeton: Princeton University Press, 1991), chapter 1.

24. Dubos, *White Plague,* 69. See also see F. B. Smith, *The Retreat of Tuberculosis, 1850–1950* (London: Croom Helm, 1988).

25. John Harley Warner, *The Therapeutic Perspective: Medical Practice, Knowledge, and Identity in America, 1820–1885* (Cambridge: Harvard University Press, 1986), 58.

26. Frederick L. Hoffman, "Mortality from Respiratory Diseases in Dusty Trades (Inorganic Dusts)," United States Department of Labor, Bureau of Labor Statistics, *Bulletin No. 231* (Washington D.C.: General Printing Office, June 1918), 30.

27. George W. Norris, "The Differential Diagnosis Between Incipient Pulmonary Tuberculosis, Healed Cavities, and Non-Tuberculosis Fibrosis," *New York Medical Journal* 80 (July 16, 1904): 103.

28. Ludwig Teleky, *History of Factory and Mine Hygiene* (New York: Columbia University Press, 1948), 199.

29. Correspondence, "Cause and Treatment of Consumption," *Scientific American* 90 (May 21, 1904): 403. Cf. George Rosen, *A Medical and Social Interpretation* (New York: Schuman's, 1943).

30. Heneage Gibbes, "Is the Unity of Phthisis an Established Fact?" *Boston Medical and Surgical Journal* 123 (December 25, 1890): 608.

31. Elizabeth Fee, *Disease and Discovery: A History of the Johns Hopkins School of Hygiene and Public Health, 1916–1939* (Baltimore: Johns Hopkins University Press, 1987), 19. See also Barbara Rosenkrantz, *Public Health and the State: Changing Views in Massachusetts, 1842–1936* (Cambridge: Harvard University Press, 1972), especially chapters 3, 4, and 5.

32. William Sedgewick, quoted in Fee, *Disease and Discovery,* 19.

33. This review of the pre-Progressive and European literature is based on Teleky, *History,* 196–210.

34. George Homan, "The Danger of Dust as a Cause of Tuberculosis," *Journal of the American Medical Association* 48 (March 23, 1907): 1014.

35. S. A. Knopf, "Our Duties Toward the Consumptive Poor," *Charities* 6 (February 2, 1901): 76.

36. Editorial, *Charities* 3 (November 18, 1899): 3. See also State of Connecticut, *Report of the Special Commission Appointed to Investigate Tuberculosis* (Hartford: 1908), 40.

37. "Consumption Widespread," *Charities* 3 (June 17, 1899): 9.

38. Graham Taylor, "The Industrial Viewpoint," *Charities and the Commons* 16 (May 5, 1906): 205.

39. Lillian Brandt, "Hygienic, Social, Industrial and Economic Aspects," *Charities and the Commons* 21 (November 7, 1908): 198. See also Livingston Farrand, "Prevention of Tuberculosis," *Charities and the Commons* 19 (November 16, 1907): 1065–1066, and Farrand, "To Check the Ravages of Consumption," *Charities and the Commons* 11 (September 5, 1903): 189–190, for the discussion of the implications of the progressive model of tuberculosis for education and public health campaigns.

40. See Francis Albert Rollo Russell, "The Atmosphere in Relation to Human Life and Health," quoted in Hoffman, "Mortality from Respiratory Diseases," 13.

41. An Address to the Tuberculosis Committee and to Unionists," *Charities and the Commons* 15 (January 20, 1906): 528.

42. Taylor, "The Industrial Viewpoint," 206.

43. *Annual Report of the Department of Health of the City of New York for the Years 1910–1911*, 31–33.

44. Ibid., 11.

45. Ibid., 12.

46. Ibid., 12.

47. See Duffy, *The Sanitarians;* Duffy, *A History of Public Health in New York City, 1625–1866* (New York: Russell Sage Foundation, 1968); and Duffy, *A History of Public Health in New York City, 1866–1966* (New York: Russell Sage Foundation, 1974). See also Leavitt, "'Typhoid Mary' Strikes Back," 608–629.

48. Charles Rosenberg and Janet Golden, eds., *Framing Disease: Studies in Cultural History* (New Brunswick, N.J.: Rutgers University Press, 1992), xiii.

49. Ibid., xxii.

50. See Charles Rosenberg, "What Is an Epidemic? AIDS in Historical Perspective," reprinted in Charles Rosenberg, *Explaining Epidemics and Other Studies in the History of Medicine* (New York: Cambridge University Press, 1992), 278–292.

51. David Rosner, *A Once Charitable Enterprise: Hospitals and Health Care in Brooklyn and New York, 1885–1915* (Princeton: Princeton University Press, 1986).

I

Breeding Grounds
for Disease

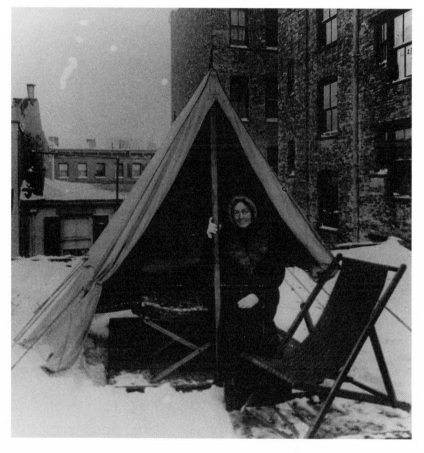

Fighting TB on the roof. Undated photograph, c. 1890s. The Jacob Riis
Collection, Museum of the City of New York.

Infectious disease outbreaks were an important cause of death throughout the early colonial period, yet, in the nineteenth century, epidemics of yellow fever, cholera, and infant diarrheal diseases played a special role in confirming the apparent disintegration of the urban environment. Although these diseases did not dramatically affect the overall rates during the century, specific communities were profoundly affected as men and women, feeble elderly, and helpless children were dramatically carried away by sudden onslaughts of intestinal diseases such as cholera or high fevers of unknown origin. In poorer communities, the toll of an epidemic was often profound; in wealthier neighborhoods, some outbreaks went virtually unnoticed.

Despite the obvious relationship between poverty and disease, there was tremendous confusion as to what particular aspect of poverty accounted for the high death and incidence rates. In the rapidly developing nineteenth-century city, it became clear that impure water, crowding, poor housing, spoiled food, and other environmental conditions were contributing factors. Especially during moments of crisis, however, some sought to focus attention on personal hygiene or child-care practices as the prime culprits causing disease. The differing explanations for high disease rates had profound implications for prevention planning. Environmental emphasis implied the need for massive social investment or changed social and economic relationships, but the emphasis on personal hygiene placed responsibility for disease on the poor and sick themselves.

Gretchen Condran opens this volume with a discussion of the overall contribution to mortality of nineteenth-century epidemic disease, pointing out the widely varied impact of disease outbreaks on different communities. Tuberculosis was clearly the greatest contributor to overall mortality during the century, but with a demographer's eye, she notes the varying patterns of epidemics. She illustrates that death rates appeared to climb for the first two-thirds of the nineteenth century and to decline thereafter. The decline in death rates seemed to confirm for many in the city that health, within certain limits, was purchasable. Despite a lack of clarity regarding what specific bacteria was associated with which particular disease, the environmental manipulation practiced by the sanitarians appears to have been effective in bringing down disease rates in this era before modern bacteriology.

In the next chapter, Elizabeth Blackmar looks at housing, an aspect of the nineteenth-century health crisis that nearly every responsible party agreed was central to any solution. She points out that health reformers sometimes had contradictory roles: they served as protectors of the public's health, generally advocating regulation, but they rarely tried to challenge broader social relationships between tenant and landlord as the city's housing market developed. The creation of a market for housing in New York sometimes worked against the creation of a healthy environment for the poor. In fact, the housing market sometimes benefited from the identification of some neighborhoods as healthy and others as diseased. Reviewing the shifting legal doctrines that affected the regulation of public and private space, she points out that "preserving public health entailed setting limits on how people could use their property." This, in turn, fostered contention over who had the right to set those limits. The creation of a housing market built around the value that "access to health depended primarily on personal ability to pay for a healthy environment" meant that health and wealth went hand in hand with better neighborhoods. Conversely, the presence of high disease rates in some neighborhoods served to raise the value of housing in healthier areas. Traditional ideas regarding personal responsibility for disease took on new meanings as market relations inverted cause and effect. The poor and diseased victims of the bifurcated housing market were presented as the cause of housing disintegration.

The third essay outlines the experience of immigrants arriving into the crowded tenements of New York and their encounters with their new environment. Alan Kraut begins by reminding us that every generation of newcomer has been presented as the cause, rather than the victim, of the diseases from which it suffers. He then goes on to describe the experience of immigrants, faced by mistrust, threatened by deportation if ill with trachoma, and scared by the imposing authority of the state as represented by the Ellis Island immigration experience. In his story, polio, tuberculosis, and other infectious diseases were "identified" as apparently specific to one or another ethnic group: Italians were predisposed to polio; Jews were stigmatized as a tubercular people. In his cases Kraut looks at the nativist uses of disease as a means of isolating, labeling, and blaming its victims. Although different immigrant groups responded to disease by building sanitariums and hospitals for their brethren, public services sometimes appeared bent on criminalizing the diseased by removing the ill from sight.

GRETCHEN A. CONDRAN

Changing Patterns of Epidemic Disease in New York City

Most nineteenth-century New Yorkers had a clear understanding of the word *epidemic*. It was not simply a metaphor but a grim and frightening reality. Although always high, mortality rates soared in some years because of diseases that in other years were either entirely absent or present only in much smaller numbers. In 1798, nearly 800 deaths from yellow fever increased the death toll for the year by nearly 50 percent.[1] More than 5,000 residents of New York died of cholera in 1849.[2] Smallpox killed only 26 of the city's inhabitants in 1868, but caused 920 deaths four years later.[3] The numbers of deaths attributed to typhus and typhoid or to diphtheria and croup increased and decreased with some regularity. Such events were by no means limited to New York City; for example, nearly a quarter of Philadelphia's fifty thousand people contracted yellow fever in 1793, and about four thousand of them died. Because both the numbers of epidemics and the deaths attributed to them increased throughout the eighteenth century and for the first three-quarters of the nineteenth, these years have been described as the period of great epidemics.[4]

Labeling an historical period in terms of its mortality characteristics may be particularly appropriate. The changes in mortality that accompanied the process of industrialization and urbanization during the nineteenth and the early twentieth centuries profoundly affected individuals' lives and the organization of society. The accumulation of populations in large cities in the United States, exemplified most dramatically in its largest city, New York, radically altered disease patterns. Large cities were the sites first of rising and extremely high mortality levels and major epidemics, and then of declines in death rates. The transition from high to low mortality was a widespread phenomenon, occurring in much of Europe and in Canada, the United States, New Zealand, and Australia.[5] The exact timing of the shift, uncertain because data are scarce prior to the mid-nineteenth century, especially outside large cities, probably varied somewhat from place to place, but the main features of the change were general.

All contemporary and historical studies underline the sharp differences between mortality in rural and urban areas. Rural mortality rates were probably declining by the end of the eighteenth or beginning of the nineteenth century in most of the early industrializing countries, and as long as these nations remained overwhelmingly rural, overall mortality trends reflected rural mortality conditions. Cities, on the other hand, posed new threats to health and longevity. The decline in national mortality levels was alternatively attenuated, interrupted, or reversed by both a growth in the number of densely populated, high-mortality cities and a rise in mortality in these cities during the first half of the nineteenth century. By the end of that century, the more general and complete reporting of deaths indicates rapidly declining mortality even in the nation's largest cities. Urban death rates fell so rapidly during the first three decades of the twentieth century that by 1930 the inhabitants of large cities enjoyed a life expectancy comparable to that in the less densely populated countryside and longer than had been recorded previously in human history.[6]

Epidemic diseases were a prominent aspect of the high mortality that characterized nineteenth-century cities. They were differentiated from other diseases like tuberculosis and the diarrheal diseases of the young by their sudden and unexpected occurrence and their geographic and temporal limits.[7] Outbreaks of epidemic disease could strike one city or only a few cities at any given time. Even within a city, epidemics were often limited to a circumscribed area. They were temporally specific events; contemporaries constructed well-defined beginnings and endings for each epidemic. As a consequence, epidemics elicited widespread fear and demanded both explanations and responses on the part of individuals, government agencies, and other social institutions. In contrast, endemic diseases, even the omnipresent tuberculosis, were likely to be defined as natural and accepted as unavoidable.[8]

Epidemics always evoked fear and panic, but the specific responses to them ranged widely by time, place, and the social condition of those who had to live through them. The well-to-do left the city of Philadelphia in 1793 at the first threat of yellow fever; the poor remained behind and warded off disease with camphor, vinegar, or tobacco. Meanwhile, the city's College of Physicians argued over what course to take and finally included in its list of recommendations that citizens should avoid infected persons, intemperance, and drafts. The city government cleaned the streets, provided an airy hospital for the stricken poor, burned gunpowder, and banned the tolling of church bells to mark a death because the sound was thought to lower the spirits of both the sick and the well.[9] Cholera also elicited widely varying responses.[10] Boards of health were quickly formed to design a response in many cities, and quarantine laws that had been largely neglected were hastily if casually enforced. Theaters, schools, and businesses were closed, and in some cases became emergency hospitals to accommodate the indigent sick. In at least one instance—in Chester, Pennsylvania, in 1832—infected persons were reported to have been murdered. Beyond immediate measures to combat the spread of illness and death, the orphaned, the widowed, and those thrust into poverty by an epidemic's effect on commerce demanded municipal support.

Because measures taken against epidemics were administratively incoherent and often short-lived—committees and boards of health appeared and disappeared, law enforcement tightened and waned—their immediate efficacy and their long-run effects are difficult to assess.[11] Regardless of the activities directed against them, epidemics always came to an end, and the urgent commitment to clean streets, quarantine ships, or isolate patients ended with them. Nonetheless, the responses to epidemics provide insight into the complex social context in which they occurred, a context that was undoubtedly altered by the demands that epidemics made on municipal governments, the medical establishment, and individual citizens. New York's history certainly illustrates this pattern of halting, inconsistent, yet cumulative change.

EPIDEMIC DISEASE IN NEW YORK CITY

The crude death rates for the city of New York from 1804 to 1930 shown in figure 1 illustrate a pattern of mortality change that New York shared with other large and growing cities. Although variations in the quality of the data and shifts in the age composition of New York City's population over time affected the observed mortality levels, both the trends in mortality and the large fluctuations in the death rates from year to year are accurately represented by the figure.[12]

Each of the high-mortality years in figure 1 can be explained by unusually

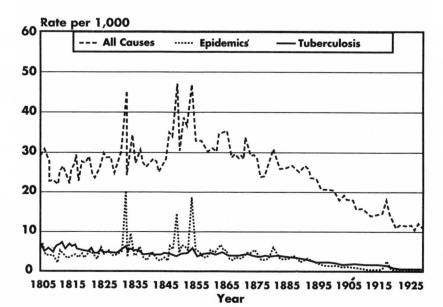

Figure 1. Death Rates, New York City, 1804 to 1930
All Causes, Epidemic Diseases, and Tuberculosis

large numbers of deaths from a particular epidemic disease. Table 1 contains a list of major outbreaks of epidemic disease in New York City from 1798 to 1918. Cholera dominated the first half century, while smallpox added to the epidemic death toll. Although an important source of the more familiar and somewhat less dramatic incursions of high mortality in the eighteenth century, and still cited as a threat in the early nineteenth, yellow fever contributed relatively few deaths after 1800. Typhus and typhoid account for the 1847 peak. Smallpox contributed most to the peaks of mortality after the 1866 cholera epidemic. Influenza and cerebrospinal meningitis were perceived as epidemics by the late nineteenth century and became important sources of exceptionally high mortality after the turn of the twentieth century, although changes in their classification may have contributed a great deal to the increase in deaths attributed to them.[13]

Neither the specific diseases that dominated particular points in time nor the yearly pattern of epidemic mortality can be easily explained. Both nineteenth-century and recent studies have shown close connections between cholera and the quality of a city's water supply. Similarly, there was undoubtedly some association between yellow fever and the extent and subsequent drainage of marshland (with the accompanying effect on local mosquito populations). Because general changes in living standards, the interconnections between causes of death, and the changes in diseases themselves probably played a role in the rise and fall of each of these diseases, it is impossible to assess the importance of any particular factor.

Cholera and yellow fever defined the practical and emotional meaning of epidemics during the late eighteenth and early nineteenth centuries. Virtually no deaths from these two diseases were recorded in the nonepidemic years. They arrived suddenly, ran their course in a matter of months, and then returned some years later with little or no warning. The symptoms of these two diseases were so spectacular that survivors were not likely to forget the experience of an epidemic. Diarrhea, spasmodic vomiting, and painful cramps followed by dehydration, cyanosis, and sudden death were characteristic of cholera.[14] Those afflicted with yellow fever suffered from fever and associated headache, nausea, clamminess, weak pulse, and the identifying yellowish cast to the complexion. As with cholera, death often ensued within the day or even within hours of the onset of symptoms.[15] That a person could be well in the morning and dead before nightfall, a stark contrast to the lingering illness associated with many endemic diseases like tuberculosis, added to the fear and panic that accompanied these epidemic diseases.

The prevalence of both cholera and yellow fever varied across the city. The New York City Board of Health noted that the "cholera fields" delineated in certain areas of the city were invariably characterized by "crowded and filthy dwellings, mostly tenant housing of the poorer classes; filthy streets, gutters and courts, obstructed and faulty house and privy sewerage, and a foul con-

Table 1. Years of Unusually Large Numbers of Deaths from Selected Epidemic Diseases, 1798 to 1918

Year	Epidemic disease	Number of deaths from disease	Percentage of excess deaths from disease
1798	Yellow fever	714	55.5
1804	Smallpox	199	10.6
1805	Yellow fever	270	13.5
1822	Yellow fever	166	5.8
1824	Smallpox	394	10.7
1832	Cholera	3,513	54.4
1834	Cholera	971	12.7
1834	Smallpox	233	2.8
1835	Smallpox	351	5.7
1847	Typhus/typhoid	1,396	10.4
1848	Smallpox	585	10.4
1848	Typhus/typhoid	953	10.4
1849	Cholera	5,071	28.9
1851	Smallpox	586	2.8
1851	Typhus/typhoid	1,103	2.8
1852	Smallpox	516	2.6
1853	Smallpox	681	3.3
1854	Cholera	2,501	10.2
1854	Smallpox	624	2.4
1864	Typhus/typhoid	1,425	2.4
1865	Smallpox	674	2.4
1865	Typhus/typhoid	1,074	2.4
1866	Cholera	1,137	4.5
1872	Smallpox	1,866	6.1
1872	Meningitis	782	6.1
1875	Smallpox	1,899	6.6
1881	Diphtheria	4,894	14.5
1887	Diphtheria	4,509	13.1
1893	Meningitis	489	.5
1901	Smallpox	410	.6
1902	Smallpox	310	.5
1904	Meningitis	1,083	.5
1905	Meningitis	1,110	.5
1906	Meningitis	600	.5
1918	Influenza	12,562	14.7

Note: The epidemics listed in table 1 are necessarily somewhat arbitrarily selected. I have used a similar table from Wilson G. Smillie, *Public Health* (New York: Macmillan, 1955), 382; a graph from the Health Department of the City of New York, *Summary of Vital Statistics* (New York, 1988); and the general cause of death listings. In general, I have included years of unusually large numbers of deaths from causes of death that were considered epidemic.

dition of privies."[16] They were coterminous with those in earlier cholera epidemics, and also, although not perfectly, with former swamplands, streambeds, and basins that were drained by surface sewers. Factors and circumstances were interrelated and varied from city to city and from disease to disease, but the geographic distribution of epidemics was fairly consistently associated with poverty.

Other diseases classified as epidemic approximated the model defined by cholera and yellow fever. The numbers of deaths from smallpox, typhoid, typhus, and later diphtheria, influenza, and meningitis were not negligible in any year, but substantially higher numbers of deaths from these diseases in some years placed them in the category of epidemic, or at least potentially epidemic, diseases. The beginnings and endings of these epidemics were less clear than in cholera or yellow fever epidemics. Public health officials consistently classified measles among the epidemic diseases, although it differed from cholera and yellow fever in both the regularity of its occurrence and its nearly exclusive threat to children.

Diseases with a strong seasonal pattern, most notably the diarrheal diseases of infants and young children, shared some characteristics with epidemic diseases. Large numbers of deaths from diarrhea occurred in the summer, but the numbers varied little from year to year and the summer peak occurred each year in every large city in the country. The extreme variation in incidence across the year suggested some association with epidemic diseases whose incidence varied across time, and diarrheal diseases of young children were classified in mid-century in the same general category with epidemic diseases; they were not generally referred to as explicitly epidemic until the end of the nineteenth century, however, when it became accepted usage to say that an epidemic of infant deaths from diarrheal diseases occurred every summer.[17]

With the exception of cholera in a handful of years, epidemic diseases accounted for a small percentage of all deaths even in epidemic years. Deaths from endemic diseases like tuberculosis, bronchitis, and pneumonia were far more important determinants of the levels of mortality at any given time. Although they rarely exacted a higher toll than endemic diseases, epidemics nonetheless altered mortality levels in an epidemic year. During the months of the 1849 cholera epidemic, the citizens of New York City experienced mortality at levels that, had they continued, would have produced an expectation of life at birth nearly fifteen years less than the approximately forty-five years implied by the mortality rates in 1844, a nonepidemic year.[18] Epidemics often changed the age pattern as well as the level of mortality. Cholera increased the death rates at all ages but especially those for young adults. Epidemics of diphtheria, meningitis, measles, and whooping cough, of course, added to the ranks of those who would not survive to adulthood. We cannot assess the significance of these diseases by their contribution to overall mortality alone.

They elicited such widespread fear and response that their psychological and political impact is only partially measured by the resulting death rate.

THE MORTALITY TRANSITION IN NEW YORK CITY

The crude death rates shown in figure 1 mask a great deal of variation in the timing and rate of mortality change by age and cause of death. In 1840, approximately 190 of every 1,000 infants born in New York City never reached their first birthdays; in 1870 that figure had passed 200. By 1930, however, fewer than 70 in 1,000 infants born in New York City died in the first year of life. Young adults also faced harsh mortality conditions in both 1840 and 1870—nearly one-quarter of those reaching the age of twenty would not live to thirty. Sixty years later, however, only 32 of 1,000 twenty-year-olds died before their thirtieth birthday. Although mortality rates dropped for all ages after 1870, the timing of the reduction differed by age group. Childhood mortality levels declined throughout the six decades from 1870 to 1930 but declined most rapidly between 1890 and 1900. Adult mortality remained high until after 1900, however, and for some middle-adult age groups rose between 1880 and 1890. The mortality rates of the elderly declined later than those for all other age groups; their death rates rose until the 1910–1920 decade and dropped dramatically between 1920 and 1930.

Data classified by cause of death illuminate the trends in age-specific mortality. In table 2 are the percentage contributions to the overall mortality decline from a number of causes of death in New York City for three time periods: 1840/45 to 1870; 1870 to 1900; and 1900 to 1930. The rates reported in table 2 are age-standardized death rates that remove the effects of changing age composition on mortality levels by assuming a constant age distribution over the time examined. Overall mortality levels increased between 1840/45 and 1870 but declined substantially during the two later time periods. Tuberculosis was the specific cause of death that explained the highest percentage of the decline in the age-standardized death rate for both periods of mortality decline. Tuberculosis accounted for 26 percent of the decline in mortality from 1870 to 1900 and 19.6 percent from 1900 to 1930. Smallpox played an important role in the early decline in overall mortality, but was a much less important source of decline after the turn of the twentieth century. Change in the rates of death from diphtheria and pneumonia made substantial contributions to the decline in the later period but, counter to the trend in overall mortality, actually rose slightly from 1870 to 1900. Diarrheal diseases were another important determinant of both the level of mortality and the changes in the level over time. They account for 15 percent of the decline in the age-standardized death rates shown in table 2 and were especially important to the decline in early death, accounting for nearly a quarter of the change in the infant and early childhood death rates.

Table 2. Age-standardized Mortality Rates by Selected Causes and Percentage Contribution to Overall Mortality Decline: New York City, 1840/45, 1870, 1900, and 1930

Cause of death	Central mortality rates (per 100,000)				Percentage of change explained by cause[a]		
	1840/45	1870	1900	1930	1840/45 to 1870	1870 to 1900	1900 to 1930
Diphtheria and croup	49.1	76.0	57.4	5.3	10.7	2.2	6.6
Diarrheal diseases	251.1	273.9	143.6	18.2	9.1	15.1	15.8
Epidemic meningitis	.0	63.9	25.9	3.4	25.5	4.4	2.8
Erysipelas	10.1	12.2	6.0	3.7	.8	.7	.3
Influenza	3.3	.0	17.6	11.5	-1.3	-2.9	.8
Malaria	22.4	23.8	5.1	.0	.6	2.2	.6
Measles	21.9	42.3	16.2	2.1	8.2	3.0	1.8
Pneumonia	161.1	193.5	241.7	126.6	12.9	-5.6	14.5
Scarlet fever	46.4	94.2	20.0	1.2	19.1	8.1	2.4
Smallpox	11.2	38.6	3.7	.0	10.9	4.0	.5
Tuberculosis	473.0	433.6	210.0	54.0	-15.7	25.9	19.6
Typhoid	38.8	39.3	17.5	1.0	.2	2.5	2.1
Whooping cough	32.5	30.0	11.0	3.5	-1.0	2.2	.9
Residual	1,260.6	1,310.7	992.6	743.0	20.0	36.8	31.4
Total	2,381.5	2,631.8	1,768.0	973.6	100.0	100.0	100.0

Note: Rates are standardized on the age distribution of the 1870 population. The years 1840 and 1845 were averaged, 1870, 1900, 1930 represent an average of three years around that year.

[a] A negative number indicates that the cause of death changed counter to the trend in overall mortality: that is, these causes declined from 1840/45 to 1870 and rose during the two later time periods.

The epidemic diseases in this analysis made only a minor contribution to mortality decline after 1870 but were more important determinants of the upturn in mortality during the first half of the nineteenth century. Smallpox, scarlet fever, and diphtheria/croup, together account for 40 percent of the rise in the age-standardized death rate. Assessing the role of epidemics in mortality change is problematic because the presence or absence of an epidemic at the beginning or end of a time period affects the calculated importance of a disease. The contribution of epidemic diseases to the general mortality pattern can be shown more effectively by combining the death rates from a number of epidemic diseases and tracing the change in the combined death rate over time.[19] The results of this strategy are shown in figure 1. The importance of these diseases increased markedly during the first six decades of the century and declined thereafter. The third line on figure 1 shows the course of the death rate from pulmonary tuberculosis. The obvious steady and slow decline in tuberculosis death rates for much of the nineteenth century was replaced by more rapid decline at the turn of the century, a course of change followed by many other endemic diseases as well. Although a number of endemic diseases may already have begun to decline in the first half of the nineteenth century, the increase in epidemic diseases played an important demographic role by countering that decline and producing mortality levels that were either stagnant or rising until the late nineteenth century. After that, epidemic diseases also declined, but their contribution to the transition to low mortality was overshadowed by rapid declines in the major endemic causes of death.

UNDERSTANDING MORTALITY AND MORTALITY CHANGE

Historians and demographers have explanations for the high and rising urban mortality rates in the first half of the nineteenth century, for the presence of frequent and massive epidemics, and for the subsequent dramatic decline in both. The growth of cities and the increased density and changes in population composition that such growth entailed for most of the nineteenth century are viewed as precipitating or exacerbating a series of problems affecting the health of city dwellers. Bad housing, overcrowding, contamination of food, pollution of water supplies, and inadequate sanitary facilities conspired, in this view, to shorten the lives of children and adults alike. Epidemics could be understood in similar terms. Susceptible populations crowded in large cities, and the flow of new inhabitants provided the necessary conditions for the spread of epidemic diseases through contaminated water or food, close personal contact, or insect vectors.

Scholars have debated the reasons for the dramatic decline in mortality in the late nineteenth and early twentieth centuries. Influenced by the work of English social medicine advocate Thomas McKeown and his colleagues, many attribute the general decline in mortality in early industrializing nations largely to economic growth and the improvements in nutrition that accompanied it. The decline in death rates is seen as a happy if largely unanticipated consequence of rising per capita income rather than a result of any purposive action to reduce mortality levels.[20] Empirical studies have not uniformly supported the McKeown hypothesis, and his critics have offered variables not necessarily related to income to explain mortality decline. One configuration of factors includes a series of public health activities: the building of sewers; filtration of water systems; activities of local boards of health in cleaning city streets, quarantining, inspecting, and regulating food and milk supplies; bacteriological screening of healthy carriers, and more. A second group of variables relates to individual hygiene and child-care practices, private as opposed to public health activities. Recognizing the interrelations among these variables, both demographers and historians increasingly find one-dimensional explanations of mortality change inadequate. Rather, the simultaneous change in many competing explanatory variables suggests that mortality decline resulted from complicated, sometimes locally specific interactions of many variables.

Epidemic diseases, varying a great deal across time and place and affecting large numbers of people at the same time, called for different explanations and responses than endemic diseases. The explanation was more environmental than individual; the intervention emphasized public rather than private activity. The city government responded to epidemic disease through a series of activities that changed over the course of the nineteenth century but aimed to protect the residents from epidemics by altering the environment the city provided them. The waning of epidemics by the end of the century seemed a testament to the effectiveness of this strategy. Progress could be measured by tracking the size of epidemics and the importance of infectious diseases more generally. In its 1866 report, the newly formed Board of Health claimed responsibility for controlling the cholera epidemic in that year and attributed the small number of deaths (compared to the previous cholera epidemic) to its understanding of the nature of epidemics and the activities it had undertaken to control the spread of the disease. The 1866 report concluded with the optimistic assessment "that no labors, plans, or acts of local cleansing, sanitary care, abatement of nuisances, or special disinfection to prevent the propagation of cholera, have been in vain; and more that none of these could have been omitted without great peril to the inhabitants and the commerce of the metropolis and the continent."[21] This activist response is more significant than its possible—and debatable—efficacy in New York's 1866 cholera outbreak.

The emotional and institutional response to epidemics far outweighed their significance as a source of mortality. Contemporaries no doubt overestimated the importance of the decline of epidemic diseases in the overall mortality decline and hence the importance of the measures they had taken against them. At least in part because of the presence of great epidemics, however, the structures for municipal response were in place. With the decline in epidemic diseases, they were refocused on endemic diseases. By the late nineteenth century, municipal intervention had shifted from large-scale sanitation projects to programs of education in personal hygiene, care of the home, and child care. The shift in program accommodated new etiologic ideas and the rise of scientific medicine but also coincided with the end of large-scale epidemics and the subsequent emphasis on endemic disease, understood in terms of individual lifestyle or constitution.

REMEMBERING PAST EPIDEMICS

Although cholera and yellow fever defined the word *epidemic* for nineteenth-century New Yorkers, metaphoric uses have blurred the original meaning for their late-twentieth-century counterparts. The sudden appearance of Acquired Immune Deficiency Syndrome (AIDS) in the late 1970s, however, has reminded us that infectious diseases remain a threat despite their declining importance and forty years of antibiotic treatment. A series of twentieth-century epidemics, most notably the influenza epidemic of 1918 and a number of epidemics of poliomyelitis starting in 1916, weakens the discontinuity between the nineteenth century epidemics and the AIDS epidemic of the 1980s. More than 130,000 New Yorkers contracted influenza in the fall of 1918, and 12,532 deaths were recorded from the disease, while the deaths recorded from its sequela, pneumonia, doubled to nearly 14,000. Influenza appeared suddenly in the early fall and had run its course by the middle of November.[22] Polio affected a much smaller segment of the population than influenza and consequently produced many fewer deaths. The response to polio, however, illustrates the link between nineteenth- and twentieth-century epidemics, as municipal health officials, remembering typhoid and typhus, directed preventive measures against the 1916 polio epidemic to the crowded slum areas of the city although polio was equally or more likely to affect the children of the affluent.[23] The limited nature of and successful prophylactic measures against polio coupled with the failure of influenza to recur in as virulent a form and the antibiotic treatment of pneumonia and other diseases contributed to the shared sense that the age of infectious-disease epidemics was indeed over. AIDS shatters that illusion, reminds us of the past, and invites comparison with earlier epidemics of infectious disease.

The demographic effect of AIDS on the current mortality conditions in New York City is shown in table 3. The number presented is the percentage added by AIDS to the total number of deaths in New York City from 1983 to 1988; it is directly comparable to the figures for epidemic diseases in table 1. By 1988, AIDS had added 5 percent to the total number of deaths in the city. The figures for some age groups are extremely grim. In 1988, AIDS raised the number of deaths in the male population age twenty-five to forty-four by 50 percent and added nearly 40 percent more deaths to women age twenty-five to

Table 3. Deaths from AIDS, New York City, 1983 to 1988

Year	Number of deaths	Percentage of excess deaths from AIDS[a]
1983	425	.6
1984	952	1.3
1985	1,663	2.3
1986	2,650	3.6
1987	3,159	4.3
1988	3,739	5.0

Source: Department of Health, City of New York, Summary of Vital Statistics 1988: The City of New York, (New York: Bureau of Health and Statistics and Analysis, 1988).
[a]The percentage of exess deaths is calculated using the number of deaths attributed to AIDS in the numerator and the total deaths minus the AIDS deaths in the denominator.

thirty-four.[24] Although the contribution of AIDS to the general mortality level is small compared to many, although certainly not all, epidemics in the past, we are shocked by the importance of an infectious disease to mortality conditions that have been dominated for nearly half a century by cancer, heart disease, and trauma.

As this demographic analysis shows, epidemic diseases were never as important as endemic diseases in explaining the level of mortality; deaths from tuberculosis among adults and diarrheal diseases among young children were always more important sources of mortality, even in most epidemic years. In addition, although epidemic diseases declined precipitously after 1870, they were not the leading source of mortality decline. That role was played by the major endemic diseases. Epidemic diseases were most important determinants of New York City's mortality conditions in the nineteenth century than at any time before or since, but their significance even during the period of great epidemics lay as much in the responses they elicited as in their demographic role as a source of urban mortality. Recently, AIDS has given the history of epidemics an unhappy and unexpected saliency, and as with epidemics of the past, its importance will be measured not only by its death toll but by our reaction to it.

Notes

1. *Annual Report of the Board of Health for the Year Ending December 31, 1890* (New York: Martin B. Brown Company, 1891).

2. Ibid.

3. *Annual Report of the Department of Health of the City of New York for the Years 1911–1912* (New York: Martin B. Brown Company, 1913).

4. C.-E. A. Winslow, Wilson G. Smillee, James A. Doull, and John E. Gordon, *The History of American Epidemiology* (St. Louis: C. V. Mosby, 1952), 52–73.

5. The movement from high to low mortality was only part of the general demographic transition, which involved a downward shift in fertility as well. The relationship between fertility and mortality decline was complicated at both the individual household and the aggregate population levels. Morbidity was also changing in some relation to mortality and is relevant to the topic of epidemic disease. Data on morbidity, however, are sufficiently scarce that I have used mortality as the key indicator of prevailing health conditions.

6. The more rapid decline in mortality in large cities than in smaller places has been documented in many studies, including Gretchen A. Condran and Eileen Crimmins, "Mortality Differences between Rural and Urban Areas of States in the Northeastern States, 1890–1900," *Journal of Historical Geography* 6 (1980): 179–202, and Samuel H. Preston, "Resources, Knowledge, and Child Mortality: A Comparison of the U.S. in the Late Nineteenth Century and Developing Countries Today," *Proceedings, International Population Conference, International Union for the Scientific Study of Population* 4 (June 5–12, 1985): 373–388.

7. For a description of the use of the term epidemic both historically and currently see Charles E. Rosenberg, "What Is an Epidemic? AIDS in Historical Perspective," *Daedalus* 118 (Spring 1989): 1–17.

8. Nineteenth-century etiologic notions about epidemics were reflected in their classification, along with several other causes of death, as zymotic diseases. In the early 1840s, the city inspector of New York reported not only the traditional alphabetical list of deaths by cause but also a listing of deaths categorized under a number of general headings, among them the zymotic disease category that included epidemic diseases along with diarrheal diseases and all fevers. The classification scheme at first differentiated zymotic diseases from other categories that classified the remaining diseases only generally by body site (for example, diseases of the respiratory system). Later, the classification scheme clarified the characteristics of zymotic diseases by contrasting them to a second major disease category: constitutional diseases, which included most of the leading endemic sources of mortality.

The city inspector explicitly stated the rationale for classifying deaths in Board of Alderman, *The Annual Report of the City Inspector*, Document 23 (February 1, 1851), 456: "to afford materials for an investigation of the characteristics of diseases, to ascertain under what circumstances, or in what seasons they prove most fatal; to observe what are the causes of mortality to which our citizens are most liable, and to deduce therefrom practical rules in regard to the best means of prevention."

9. J. H. Powell, *Bring Out Your Dead: The Great Plague of Yellow Fever in Philadelphia in 1793* (Philadelphia: University of Pennsylvania Press, 1949).

10. See Charles E. Rosenberg, *The Cholera Years* (Chicago: University of Chicago Press, 1962).

11. In Philadelphia, the threat of cholera in 1891 led the Board of Health to employ a large corps of disinfectors and inspectors, but when cholera failed to appear they were used to combat an outbreak of diphtheria instead. Edward T. Morman, "Scientific Medicine Comes to Philadelphia: Public Health Transformed, 1854–1899" (Ph.D. diss., University of Pennsylvania, 1986).

12. The mortality rates shown in figure 1 were calculated using the reported deaths and the estimates of the midyear population of New York City. Both the deaths and

population estimates for the years 1804 to 1890 were obtained from the *Annual Report of the Board of Health for the Year Ending December 31, 1890*. Deaths and population estimates for the period from 1891 to 1928 are from Haven Emerson, *Population, Births, Notifiable Diseases, and Deaths, assembled for New York City, New York, 1866–1938* (New York: Columbia University, Delamar Institute of Public Health, 1941). The two series are somewhat discrepant when they overlap; however, the general features of mortality change would not be altered by substituting one for the other except in the years 1866, 1867, and 1869, for which Emerson appears to have erroneously included the deaths in Brooklyn, then not part of the city, in his figures.

All figures for the years prior to 1898 refer to the old City of New York, the present boroughs of Manhattan and the Bronx. After 1898, figures are for all five boroughs. The death rates for Brooklyn, Queens, and Richmond combined were slightly lower than those for the old city; therefore, the discontinuity in the area covered by the data may have a small effect on the reported trends.

13. Epidemic meningitis was confused with typhus and a number of other epidemic diseases during the entire nineteenth century according to Wilson G. Smillie, *Public Health* (New York: Macmillan, 1955). A serious outbreak in New England was described as "spotted fever," a category that appears throughout the first half of the nineteenth century in the city inspector's reports of causes of death in New York City.

14. Rosenberg, *The Cholera Years*, 2–3.

15. Powell, *Bring Out Your Dead*, 8–9.

16. *Annual Report of the Metropolitan Board of Health* (Albany, 1866), 370.

17. See Harold Lentzner and Gretchen A. Condran, "Seasonal Patterns of Infant and Childhood Mortality in New York, Chicago, and New Orleans: 1870–1920" (Paper presented at the meetings of the Population Association of America, Boston, 1985); and Gretchen A. Condran and Harold Lentzner, "An Analysis of Excess Summer Mortality of Infants and Young Children, New York City, 1820–1920" (Paper presented at the meetings of the Population Association of America, Washington, 1991).

18. The estimates of life expectancy are made by fitting North Model Life Tables to the mortality rates calculated for each of these years. The model life tables are in Ansley J. Coale and Paul Demeny, *Regional Model Life Tables and Stable Populations* (1966; reprint, New York: Academic Press, 1983). High infant and childhood mortality have a large effect on life expectancy at birth. The expected remaining years of life for those reaching age fifteen shows about a ten-year difference between the cholera year of 1849 and the nonepidemic year of 1844.

19. The diseases included in this grouping were scarlet fever, cholera, measles, smallpox, diphtheria, croup, typhoid, typhus, influenza, yellow fever, malaria, and meningitis.

It is difficult to trace the level of mortality from even a few disease categories over time. The path between the physical cause of someone's death and its appearance in a municipal summary of vital statistics is long and involves a complex set of agreements on the part of the patient, the family, the physician certifying the death, and the city government recording it. During the nineteenth century, changes in disease concepts affected the manner of recording even many of the quite distinctive symptoms manifest in these epidemic diseases. Thus, changes in disease categories influence the disease-specific death rates calculated for different points in time. How much of the rise in the death rate from diphtheria from 1840 to 1900 resulted from an actual change in the clinical incidence of a particular set of symptoms in the population and how much resulted from a more frequent diagnosis of diphtheria is largely unknowable.

In constructing the series of death rates from epidemic diseases in figure 1, I have taken account of obvious changes in disease categorization and have included in the analysis several categories in which deaths from epidemic diseases may have been hidden in the early part of the century. The figures are thereby deliberately biased against a rise in the importance of these epidemic diseases over time, an outcome that nonetheless appears in the data for the early nineteenth century.

20. See, for example, Thomas McKeown, *The Role of Medicine: Dream, Mirage, or Nemesis?* (Princeton, N.J.: Princeton University Press, 1979).

21. *Annual Report of the Metropolitan Board of Health*, 448.

22. See causes of death, nos. 11 and 16, in Emerson, *Population, Births.*

23. Naomi Rogers, "Screen the Baby, Swat the Fly: Polio in Northeastern United States, 1916" (Ph.D. diss., University of Pennsylvania, 1986).

24. Department of Health of the City of New York, *Summary of Vital Statistics 1988: The City of New York* (New York: Bureau of Health Statistics and Analysis, n.d.).

ELIZABETH BLACKMAR

Accountability for Public Health: Regulating the Housing Market in Nineteenth-Century New York City

In the late 1850s, New Yorkers expressed alarm that their city's steadily rising mortality rate now exceeded that of Old World capitals and of all other American cities. The city's annual death rate had doubled between 1810 and 1856, a statistician reported to the state assembly, and "was greater than in any city and at any period where life was valuable enough to be numbered." That the nation's richest city should also have the poorest health seemed to contradict the utilitarian faith that progress—the realization of the greatest good for the greatest number—could be measured through rising aggregate wealth made possible by unfettered market relations.[1]

Faced with this contradiction, observers at the time offered a range of explanations for New Yorkers' abysmal health: the dramatic increase in city residents—from sixty thousand in 1800 to half a million by 1850—simply overwhelmed the city; immigrants who came through the port brought their intemperance and illnesses with them; efforts to supply clean water had been obstructed first by the corporate fraud of the Manhattan Company and then by party quarrels; indifferent, inept, or corrupt politicians failed to enforce the available health ordinances. Yet by the 1850s, public health and housing reformers had also begun to focus—in the phrase that Dr. John Griscom borrowed from the British health reformer Edwin Chadwick—on the "sanitary conditions of the laboring population" as the source of the city's poor health. In the city's wealthiest ward, one out of fifty-five people died in 1856, a mortality rate half that of the city as a whole; in the city's poorest working-class ward, the rate was one in twenty-three.[2] In the minds of health reformers, such figures established public health as a social question, one that required coming to terms with the city's deepening housing crisis. That crisis—the inadequate supply of affordable, healthy housing for working people—resulted from the intersecting relations of the city's evolving labor and housing markets.

In the early nineteenth century, New Yorkers found themselves negotiating two concepts of health in relation to the market. On the one hand, health was considered a personal characteristic, the responsibility of individuals who lived within a "private" set of social relations—contractual relations—that were placed largely beyond legal regulation. On the other hand, due in large measure to epidemics, health, from the late eighteenth century on, was increasingly regarded as a social product, a feature of the city at large. Preserving public health entailed setting limits on how people could use their property within a shared landscape, expanding the legal precept that proprietors should not use their land in such a way as to injure the interests of their neighbors. Health and housing reformers developed programs to regulate health "nuisances" in alliance with the city's businessmen, and they shared with propertied New Yorkers the confidence that they could transform the city's physical environment without transforming the underlying market relations that shaped it. Yet as "personal" household relations themselves became a matter of market exchange—contingent on the securing of wages and payment of rents—so too did conditions of health themselves come to be treated not simply as a household product or a social good but also as a commodity. That is to say, access to health depended primarily on the personal ability to pay for a healthy environment.

In defining *public* health as a social concern, reformers raised the question of who was accountable—who, as the legal scholar Arthur Miller has put it in another context, "had to answer in another place"—when thousands of people died young or lived poorly. Yet, the reasoning that supported the expansion of market relations in the nineteenth century also constrained reformers' ability to establish accountability by asking further what the improving healthiness of some New Yorkers had to do with the deteriorating health of others.

ACCOUNTABILITY: GOD, PROPERTY RIGHTS, AND PERSONAL OBLIGATION

Accountability is both a moral and a legal concept, a means of attributing blame and demanding retribution or restitution. It is a concept that assumes that bad occurrences have causes that can be explained and redressed. Of course, within religious traditions, God is both the cause of human experience and the agent of retribution. Most colonial New Yorkers regarded disease as one of God's providences over which people had little control. Sinners might answer in Hell for their violation of God's will, but divine power over human life remained unaccountable.

Even secular thinkers shared something of this fatalism. In his 1788 treatise on English common law, Sir William Blackstone identified health—alongside life, limb, bodily integrity, and security of reputation—as a natural right of free persons. No one in the eighteenth century thought government could promise good health as a blessing of liberty, however. At best, governments might prevent citizens from harming one another. Apparently Blackstone did not pay much attention to the new medical opinions of his era, for he could identify only two established fields of public law that defended people's right to health: quarantine and rules against selling adulterated food.[3] By the time he wrote, however, medical investigators in ports like New York had begun to develop theories that linked disease to the environment—particularly to vitiated air—and thus suggested a new scope of public regulation.

When New York physicians investigated yellow fever epidemics from 1790 to 1825, they identified poor waterfront neighborhoods as the "ground center of the calamity." The wharf district was "thickly inhabited, its houses generally small and badly ventilated," Dr. Jonas Smith Addams typically observed in 1791. "Many of the inhabitants were in indigent circumstances," he added, "which is a frequent cause of the want of cleanliness." Since Addams and other early sanitarians subscribed to the theory that disease originated in the atmosphere, they especially decried the lack of ventilation in the close quarters of one- or two-story wood cottages built on landfill lots. Yellow fever festered, moreover, in the poorly drained yards of these houses. In 1796, Dr. Noah Webster traced the outbreak of the epidemic to Dover Street, "which [having] been raised several feet since the buildings . . . were erected," blocked the windows of the adjacent wood houses and formed a dike that flooded the yard with contaminated water. These early medical investigators had little trouble discerning why people would live in such quarters: they could not afford to live elsewhere. The "higher price of house-rent in other parts of the city," Dr. Valentine Seaman explained in 1795, "concentrated a great proportion" of the town's poorest families in the epidemic neighborhood "and crowded them in very small confined apartments." Whereas "opulent" New Yorkers fled the city during epidemic months of August and September, the "less prudent and the more indigent remained exposed to the diseases."[4]

The doctors who investigated the source of epidemics were moving away from a providential explanation for public health and illness toward a social theory of prevention. In so doing, they directed attention not simply to the sanitary condition of the environment but also to the economic position of individual households within the city. Yet, as both Addams's and Seaman's observations suggest, their empirical studies left them caught between a belief that health rested on personal virtues—prudence and cleanliness—and a new recognition of its connection to a social condition—indigence.

At the time of these investigations, most New Yorkers continued to regard health not simply as a matter of providence but also as a measure of the personal character of individual householders. In the first instance, autonomous adults were expected to exercise prudence in taking care of themselves. Although sympathetic to the "constitutionally" weak or disabled, New Yorkers were quick to judge and condemn individuals whose behaviors—drinking alcohol, for example—placed them "at risk" of disease. Health was also thought to be the collective responsibility and property of households, a quality embedded in a set of prescribed or contractual obligations. In the eighteenth century, when houses sheltered the town's trade and domestic work, most workers lived with their employers. Masters had a duty as well as an interest in maintaining the health of apprentices, journeymen, servants, and slaves who, alongside family members, constituted the household. The labors of a mistress and her servants in maintaining a household's health were among the "in kind" goods exchanged when household workers contracted for room and board. What the medical investigators added to this assumption of house-holders' responsibility for the health of dependents was the recognition that indigent—and generally tenant—households could not control the quality of the houses they occupied. The epidemics, moreover, did not confine them-selves to the quarters of the poor. They disrupted the rhythms of trade and threatened the lives and livelihoods of the entire port.

In response to the medical investigations of yellow fever epidemics, New Yorkers began to recast the common law against "nuisances" in order to as-sign accountability for the unsanitary conditions they believed bred disease. The Anglo-American legal system built its concepts of rights and wrongs on the institution of property, the cornerstone of a well-ordered society. Within this tradition, preserving every free man's right to enjoy the benefits of private property also required striking a balance of mutual restraint. Thus, a funda-mental principle of common law held that proprietors should not use land in such a way as to injure the interests of neighbors. Even before doctors identi-fied atmospheric sources of disease, common law had defined light and fresh air as essential features of a house, attributes necessary to its enjoyment. When householders created a "nuisance"—letting a privy overflow or ne-glecting manure and garbage piles, for example—their neighbors could take the direct action of removing it.[5]

In seeking to prevent or control epidemics, the early sanitary reformers appealed to city officials to expand the reach of the eighteenth-century legal concept of "common nuisances": uses of land that could be regulated by gov-ernment because they impinged on everyone's well-being. With the support of merchants (who preferred a focus on the local environment to the theories of contagion, which, in advocating quarantine, also disrupted trade), health re-formers proposed new ordinances to eliminate the physical conditions that fed disease: to regulate and regrade the streets, fill in sunken lots, clean out refuse that accumulated in slips and wharves, and introduce clean water and sewers. In addition to extending the boundaries of districts that required "fireproof" building materials, public health ordinances proscribed burials and such nui-sance industries as tanning, bone-boiling, or butchering within the built-up areas of the city. Officials also tightened regulations governing the emptying of privies and disposal of waste and garbage. The creation of the city inspec-tor's office in 1804 institutionalized city government's responsibility for health as a public concern. So too did the Common Council's hiring of street cleaners. These early ordinances represented the efforts of elected representatives to es-tablish the conditions of a healthy environment for the city as a whole.[6]

Early health reformers and government officials alike looked upon the physical environment as the manifestation of the city's progress as well as the source of disease. Worrying about the impact of the city's rapid, unregulated growth, they sought to make proprietors accountable for how they used their land. In this view, the sources of disease—overflowing privies, foul-smelling trades in proximity to dwellings, piles of manure, dead carcasses, stagnant water, polluted wells—were extrinsic to expanding market relations, not intrinsic aspects of the housing market. If nuisances were what economists later called the "externalities" of capitalist development, the unintended and unpleasant side effects, such bad "external" effects could be limited by drawing maps and establishing a set of ground rules. Proprietors could not use land in any way they wished, but since in theory all landowners gained equally from the regulation of a shared landscape, neither did they sacrifice their more fundamental rights to control their own property.

The historian John Teaford observes that nuisance laws became the primary arena of local government action in the early nineteenth century. As such, he suggests, health concerns helped define a new republican concept of the public good. Yet the historian Hendrick Hartog emphasizes the private economic interest that underlay the invention of local government's "police power" out of the common law of nuisances. In earlier generations, rules against common nuisances aimed to maintain stability and order by preventing new uses of property that disrupted "a fixed, customary order."[7] The new ordinances, by contrast, both accommodated and promoted the changes brought about by market relations, particularly the rise of a speculative housing market. Whatever the benefits to public health—and some historians think they were limited—laws banning cemeteries, wandering pigs, or ash heaps from the built-up town made some areas of the city more attractive for builders and thus encouraged higher levels of investment. The new ordinances, in effect, recast government's traditional obligation to protect private property by redefining "protection": securing property rights would entail government taking a new interest not simply in sanitary conditions but also in the "highest and best use" of land, thereby establishing the private right to the use and benefit of property as a right to profit within the capitalist economy.

The implications of the selective identification of the public good with land use regulation that enhanced property rights (and values) can be seen by comparing this development to the shifts in the doctrine of contract law, the other field of market relations that raised the question of accountability for the health of city residents. Whatever the new theories of environmental—and hence social—causes of disease in the city, most New Yorkers in the early republic still believed that health depended on the actions of individual householders. Yet the simultaneous development of wage labor and rental housing in the late eighteenth century was also altering customary definitions of the personal obligation of employers to workers and of proprietors to tenants.

A new generation of employers, who paid nonresident journeymen hourly wages, had no obligation for workers' maintenance and well-being. Landlords who collected those wages as rents had no responsibility to guarantee the quality of the domestic quarters they rented out. These contractual relations were intrinsic to the market, and in contrast to the application of nuisance law to regulate the specific uses of city property, judges were moving the doctrine of contracts away from evaluating the substance, fairness, or consequences of such market exchanges.

In the eighteenth century, legal historian Morton Horwitz has argued, contractual relations were open to scrutiny on the grounds of fairness of exchange. But the emerging legal doctrine of contracts held that judges and juries should regard and enforce all contracts simply on the basis of the agreement struck between buyers and sellers. Employers were not liable to their workers or accountable to the public, for example, if they maintained unhealthy or dangerous *working* conditions; once a person had agreed to the terms of employment, he or she accepted any risks to health that arose on the job. Common law, moreover, had long held that responsibility for the maintenance of rented quarters fell not on the landlord but on the tenant. By the mid-nineteenth century, judges were reinforcing this doctrine by applying the contract rule of *caveat emptor* ("buyer beware") to rental housing. "A bad smell in the pantry, a kitchen being too hot with the stove in it, bad smells from the front window, a stagnant pond of water near the place, bad smell from fish, vermin in the bedrooms were all matters that might have given some trouble to eradicate," a judge ruled in a typical case, "but none of them can be held sufficient to relieve the tenant from liability" for rent or require the landlord to correct them. Accountability within contractual relations thus rested primarily with the parties' obligation to look after their own interests before entering into an exchange. Whether as wage-workers or as tenants, individuals assumed the risks of their own relations with others.[8]

The legal doctrines governing common nuisances on the one hand and contractual relations on the other set limits for how New Yorkers addressed the problems of public health in the first half of the nineteenth century. The market was said to operate through invisible and ostensibly neutral laws of supply and demand. If vaguely sanctioned market relations of the society as a whole rather than the actions of particular proprietors organized the life (and deaths) of the city, no one person could be held answerable for encroachments on what Blackstone had articulated as an individual's rights to health. City officials could forbid certain land uses and require proprietors to perform certain duties. But government could not intervene in contractual relations that determined the conditions of work, the distribution of housing, or, indeed, the marketing of health itself as a commodity.

Even in the eighteenth century, the provision of health had assumed aspects of a commodity, a physical attribute of housing and a product of domestic labor that could be assigned a cash value and exchanged. In boarding houses, for example, landladies generally charged extra for nursing a sick tenant. The late-eighteenth-century health reformers who mapped the correspondence of disease and poverty observed that health carried a price tag; yet they also regarded the poor families living in the city's worst housing as exceptions within their society, not as harbingers of the future. And they believed that new city ordinances could eliminate the vitiated atmosphere and contaminated water that most directly endangered health. By the 1820s, however, far from being an isolated condition, poverty represented the permanent outcome of contractual relations between the city's laboring families and their employers and landlords. And the value assigned to health, produced in a domestic set-ting, had become one of the selling points of domestic property as well as of domestic labor. Light and air could not be easily insured by defending a household from neighbors' nuisances, but these features of housing could be purchased or leased. Thus, despite the flurry of ordinances, securing health was becoming a matter of individual households establishing priorities for spending their own money. If epidemics helped shape a consciousness of the city as a shared environment and the "public's" right to health, fear of epi-demics also propelled the organization of a bifurcated housing market. Gov-ernment policy, viewing public health as coterminous with economic development, not only tolerated but promoted the formation of this class-divided housing market that would, in turn, push reformers to focus on the housing crisis as the source of the city's health crisis.

HEALTH AND THE FORMATION OF THE BIFURCATED HOUSING MARKET

During the yellow fever and cholera epidemics of the late eighteenth and early nineteenth centuries, the most common means of defending the right to health was to look out for oneself. Those families who could afford to, got out of town. Those who could not remained behind to nurse the sick and bury the dead. City officials compensated for the failure of their preventive measures by evacuating pestilent neighborhoods and providing temporary housing north of the port. But such dramatic government initiatives during emergencies be-lied the prevailing belief that health was primarily a measure of an indi-vidual's and a households' virtue and habits—the qualities of disciplined character that, within republican thought, represented the means to self-pro-tection. Those who properly valued health would take care to maintain a clean, well-ventilated dwelling.

In the early decades of the nineteenth century, then, Manhattan's housing market developed above all else as a market in health. The concentration of yellow fever epidemics in the wharf district altered the way New Yorkers valued housing and particular locations. The recurrent epidemics must have come as a sore shock, for example, to the prominent merchant families who had in the late 1780s and 1790s invested their fortunes in new mansions in the heart of the port. Removing their offices and counting rooms from their houses to wharf-front stores, the proprietors of Bowling Green, State Street, and lower Broadway had nonetheless placed a premium on maintaining dwellings close to the centers of trade, as well as to one another's households. However convenient for business, the prime location of these downtown dwellings rendered them all the more vulnerable to disease in August and September. In 1799, Elizabeth Bleeker, who lived on lower Broadway, was shocked that a black man who was dying of yellow fever "came up our alley and laid himself down on the ground"; in August four years later she noted in her diary that her brother had removed his family from Water Street because "several persons have died near him with the fever." The wealthiest families annually left the city for country homes and resorts; during the 1805 epidemic, more than one-third of the city's residents moved out of downtown in late summer.[9]

The new demand for dwellings beyond the wharf district spurred speculative construction in the early decades of the century. In 1807, a "small genteel family" advertised its desire for domestic quarters and typically noted that "the neighborhood must be respectable and in a healthy part of the city where it would not be necessary to remove in the event of the fever." Builders responded to these concerns by featuring "healthiness of situation" in their advertisements for new houses, and they found a ready market among merchant and professional families who sought to insulate themselves from the threat of fever. Although expensive, a new dwelling north of Chambers Street might save a family the cost of suspending business and paying for temporary domestic quarters two or three months a year.[10]

In increasing the allocation of family income to new dwellings and housekeeping, propertied and middle-class New Yorkers elaborated their ideas about "the home" as the center for both morality and health, the two inextricably linked. Caring for the sick, of course, had long been a domestic labor. But domestic literature in the 1830s and 1840s, which promulgated new standards of housekeeping, underscored the association of health and housing and helped define the features of new dwellings—their siting and their utilities— as necessities rather than luxuries. (Indeed, the nineteenth century's spiraling costs of health care could be measured not in the costs of technology, science, or doctors but in the new levels of capital investment in housing.) By the 1840s, writers like Catharine Beecher were stressing the importance of well-designed houses in order for women to fulfill their domestic responsibilities in caring for family health and morals. In defining the values of home life in opposition to the market, writers like Beecher helped obscure the connection between the two.[11]

The speculative production of healthy and respectable neighborhoods beyond the port, however, introduced a new dynamic to the housing market.

Artisan families had first moved to the port's periphery to escape the high rents of prime commercial land in lower Manhattan. Often leasing land from a rentier, they initially built inexpensive two-story wood and brick-front houses and shops on the Lower East Side in the vicinity of the shipyards or on the West Side along Hudson Street and in Greenwich Village. As wealthier families devoted a substantial portion of their incomes to purchasing dwellings in neighborhoods north of Chambers Street, land and housing prices soared. So did rents. Through the building boom of the 1820s and early 1830s, builders and developers produced the largest number of new dwellings for the most lucrative and economically secure market: wealthy and middle-class families. Substantial brick or stone townhouses offered not only roomy, well-ventilated interiors but new utilities as well. Although frequently shared by two families and their servants, blocks of "single-family" row-houses formed the city's respectable neighborhoods west of Broadway.[12]

By feeding the speculative land market between Chambers and Fourteenth streets and establishing builders' and developers' new expectations for the rate of profit from construction, propertied New Yorkers' demands for new dwellings in the years 1800 to 1840 established the connection between one group's pursuit of healthy living conditions and the deterioration of the living conditions of others. Although small builders also erected new brick-front and wood dwellings for artisan households east of Broadway, fewer and fewer wage-earning families could afford to pay rent for an entire house. While single journeymen and day laborers found domestic accommodations in the city's proliferating boarding houses, working-class families went to housekeeping in former artisan houses subdivided for three or more families. Through subdivision, boarding houses and tenant houses emerged from within the city's oldest housing stock; once a neighborhood had been socially "devalued" through the concentration of tenant and boarding houses, investors avoided building new dwellings that cost more than the neighborhood market could bear. The builders' main concession to the city's growing number of working-class families before 1830 was to anticipate further subdivision by introducing three-story rather than two-story rental houses east of Broadway, thereby increasing the space that could be subdivided into apartments when landlords sought more tenants.

By the late 1820s, the city's new class geography was apparent in the contrasting density and quality of housing stock in wealthy and working-class districts. As Charles Rosenberg and others have noted, evangelical and temperance reformers who visited the poor to distribute religious tracts in the late 1820s and 1830s saw a danger to the city's health and morals in old and closely built tenant neighborhoods. Yet they were ambivalent about where to place the blame for the deteriorating conditions. Moral reform, after all, required that individuals take personal responsibility for the habits of cleanliness that signaled piety and produced health, and many commentators blamed poor housing conditions on Irish immigrants who did not follow the codes of Protestant rectitude. Doctor Jonas Addams, however, was not the last health reformer to attribute poor housekeeping habits themselves to "indigent circumstances." By the 1840s, John Griscom would judge inattention to cleanliness a symptom of poverty—"demoralization"—rather than its cause.[13]

Whatever the assessment of cause and effect with respect to poverty and cleanliness, the continuing identification of health with morality in *housing* circumscribed the vocabularies of reform when it came to explaining why working-class living conditions were growing worse. In the 1830s, as rents continued to soar with the economic boom that accompanied the opening of the Erie Canal, even middle-class New Yorkers complained that the provision of housing was governed by a "spirit of avarice." They were reluctant, however, to condemn that same spirit in other arenas of the economy. In 1834, the city inspector, noting that "some cause should be assigned for the increase of deaths beyond the increase of population," merged moral and market explanations. No cause "appears so prominent as that of intemperance, and the crowded and filthy state in which a great proportion of our population live, and apparently, without being sensible of their situation," he observed. He then went on to echo a widespread complaint by adding, "We have serious cause to regret that there is [sic] in our city so many mercenary landlords, who contrive in what manner they can stow the greatest number of human beings in the smallest space." There were two sides to the formation of the city's housing market, and the quality of housing New Yorkers could afford to buy or rent was also determined by what they could earn in wages. Despite the mobilization of a citywide labor movement in the 1830s, "mercenary" employers—or the conditions of the wage relation itself—did not figure in the health reformers' attribution of responsibility for rising poverty or early death.[14]

In any case, aldermen in the early 1830s were less worried about the growing poverty, immorality, or mortality of wage-earning families than about promoting new improvements that would enhance New York's status as the nation's economic capital. They enthusiastically supported the differentiation in housing standards by creating private residential squares like Gramercy Park and granting tax breaks to developers for landscaping public spaces like Union Square. In subsidizing elite residential development, officials paid lip service to the health benefits of these open spaces, but they seemed more impressed by the benefits to real estate values. Indeed, the republican concept of a public whose good lay in preventing proprietors from injuring the interests of their neighbors was rapidly giving way to a new abstract and utilitarian public whose greatest good could be measured by the aggregate figures of rising land values, population growth, and increasing capital investment in industry. Aldermen recognized that their policies led to the displacement of poorer tenants, but they saw no direct link between improvement and deterioration. "The exceeding rapid increase of our population, and the measures which have been taken to lay out and form public squares," a typical report observed, "have so much enhanced the value of lots in their vicinity as to render it desirable for persons of lesser means to turn their attention to situations somewhat more removed . . . where lots can be purchased at such a moderate rate as to come within their means."[15] Yet with the de-skilling of crafts and the expansion of the waged labor market, proprietorship was permanently giving way to tenancy for more and more people "of lesser means"; they had little choice but to move into the already crowded rental quarters of subdivided houses.

Given the utilitarian perspective in business and governmental circles, the growing problems of public health registered most strongly when the aggregate figures of rising mortality rates, exacerbated by the 1832 cholera epidemic, threatened the city's commercial reputation. Aldermen, debating the introduction of the Croton aqueduct, stressed that Philadelphia had gained a competitive edge by solving its water (and thus its health and fire) problems. It was the New York fire insurance companies that most aggressively campaigned for a new water system.[16] The construction of the Croton aqueduct satisfied demands for a clean water source that health reformers had been making for nearly three decades. Yet in its first fifty years the new water system and the sewers that followed reached a selective public, for the rising costs of housing were not matched by increased income for the majority of the city's families.

Building owners had to pay for the introduction of water pipes and fixtures to their houses as well as a tax for use. Not surprisingly, many landlords, calculating that they would not be able to pass this expense on to tenants, ignored the opportunity. Landlord William Gibbons, who owned both middle-class dwellings and multifamily tenant houses throughout the city, resisted the introduction of Croton water: "I will not contribute anything toward it or undertake to furnish water for any tenant," he informed his agent just after the new system opened.[17] Finding he had no choice but to pay the general water tax, Gibbons nonetheless introduced pipes only to houses with middle-class tenants and then raised their rents. Far from regarding himself as acting from immoral or "mercenary" motives, Gibbons thought he followed the sound investment practice of any sensible capitalist.[18]

Even landlords who might want to introduce running water or plumbing were constrained by the location of street pipes, and here city policy often ratified landowners' strategies for maintaining what they judged a satisfactory rate of return on their investments. Since landowners paid assessments for introducing sewers, for example, aldermen usually awaited their petitions before taking action. Sewers, Gibbons once again protested to his agent, "are an unhealthy arrangement and should be avoided at all times if possible. A street can be kept in better order by [washing] the accumulated matter on the surface of the ground—than by depositing it in a sewer." When neighboring proprietors successfully petitioned for a sewer on Spruce Street where he owned houses, Gibbons concluded, "if I am assessed for construction and made to pay, the payment entitles me to any advantage the sewer offers," particularly the advantage of raising rents.[19] But where wage-earning tenants could not afford to pay, landowners and public officials were slow to act. In 1857 the Association for Improving the Condition of the Poor (AICP) complained that only 138 miles of pipes had been constructed in 500 miles of streets, leaving "nearly three-fourths of the city, including some of the densely populated and filthy portions, without sewers."[20]

The introduction of water, plumbing, and gas lighting all contributed to a redefinition of housing standards in the 1840s and 1850s and reinforced middle-class New Yorkers' conviction that sanitation and ventilation were the keys to health. Yet the very improvement of living conditions for the city's more prosperous households continued to push up land values and rents and highlighted the absolute and relative deterioration of tenant-houses, where hydrants in the yard and old-fashioned privies remained common through the second half of the nineteenth century. At the end of the century, despite another fifty years of sanitary and housing reform, more than half of Manhattan's families still relied on privies rather than toilets.[21] The housing market would deliver sanitation only to those who could afford to pay for it.

THE HOUSING CRISIS AND HEALTH REFORM: SELECTIVE ACCOUNTABILITY

By the 1840s, medical opinion, domestic literature, and the housing market reinforced New Yorkers' identification of health with the quality of housing. But it was the collapse of construction following the Panic of 1837 that most directly prompted New Yorkers to link the city's rapidly rising mortality rates with an emerging housing crisis. The panic brought an abrupt halt to the construction boom of the 1830s; with builders declaring bankruptcy and thousands of New Yorkers unemployed, landlords responded to hard times by further subdividing houses, adding wood rear-houses, and renting out cellars to the poorest tenants. Against this backdrop of economic depression, the physician and city inspector John Griscom launched a new phase of sanitary reform in his 1842 report when he singled out "the crowded condition, with insufficient ventilation" of dwellings as "first among the most serious causes of disordered general health."[22]

Griscom sought to assure his readers that there was nothing inherently unhealthy about New York City's climate and physical location; he stressed that rising mortality reflected the vulnerability of the city's growing number of poor immigrants. "Living with their acquaintance awhile in crowded apartments, in cellars, in crumbling tenements, and narrow courts and streets, and upon food poor in quality, and stinted in quantity, they are peculiarly exposed to inroads of disease, and none more than consumption." Drawing on the reports of tract missionaries and his own observations, Griscom warned that nearly 34,000 people were living in the 1,459 dark and damp cellar dwellings and 1,727 courts and rear-houses. (He might also have noted that as many as 40,000 New Yorkers were without any shelter that year; they were identified as "indigent lodgers" in the station houses.) In Griscom's eyes, housing conditions exposed the interconnectedness of the environmental, moral, and social dimensions of disease. "The over-crowded state of many tenements, and the want of separate apartments, are prolific sources of moral degradation, and physical suffering," he wrote. Multiple families living in close quarters not only produced a vitiated atmosphere, but also "an indifference to the common decencies of life, and a disregard of the sacred obligations of moral propriety, which result in a depressing effect upon the physiological energies, and powerfully heighten the susceptibility to, aggravate the type, and render more difficult the cure, of diseases among them." Not only did early death follow, but such conditions also sapped the capacity of individuals to take responsibility for their own lives and the well-being of their families.[23]

In many respects, Griscom's report and his pamphlet on the sanitary condition of the laboring population, which followed two years later, built on the theories and recommendations that city inspectors and sanitarians had been making for three decades. Like his predecessors, he called for the elimination of common nuisances, regulation of noxious industries, cleaning of streets, and introduction of clean water and sewers. But Griscom also redirected attention from the sanitary conditions of wharves, streets, and sunken lots to the interior conditions of tenant houses; taking the fire laws as his model, he proposed a new reach of public regulation. "If there is any propriety in the law regulating the construction of buildings in reference to fire," he argued, "equally proper would be one respecting the protection of the inmates from the pernicious influence of badly arranged houses and apartments." Griscom urged that the definition of public nuisance "be extended to the correction of interior conditions of tenements when dangerous to health and life. The latter should be regarded with as much solicitude as the prosperity of citizens."[24]

Like his predecessors, however, Griscom faced the problem of proposing a remedy for physical ills that arose from the social relations that had produced prosperity for some New Yorkers and new extremes of poverty for others; such a remedy required deciding who was accountable. Griscom took the trouble to investigate the economics of the housing market, but his conclusions remained circumscribed by his own understanding of the ground rules of his society. Although he denounced the "system of tenantage to which large numbers of the poor are subjected," he focused on the "merciless inflation and extortion of the *sublandlord*," the middlemen of New York City's tiered tenant system. "A house, or a row, or a court of houses is hired by some person of the owner, on a lease of several years, for a sum that will yield a fair interest on the costs," he reported. "The owner is thus relieved of the great trouble incident to the changes of tenants and the collection of rent. His income is sure from one individual, is obtained without annoyance or oppression on his part. It then becomes the object of the lessee to make and save as much as possible, with his adventure, sometimes to enable him to purchase the property in a short time."[25] Griscom correctly described the system of subtenancy that had arisen with the subdivision of rental houses, but he absolved the city's rentiers and primary landlords of responsibility by endorsing their profits—the "fair interest on the costs"—while denouncing villainous sublandlords' "extortions." Working-class sublandlords operated under the constraint of the rent they owed the chief landlord, who measured a "fair" return on an investment by comparing it to alternative outlets for capital. For Griscom to have gone further and challenged the right of rentiers to profit from slum housing would have been to alienate a political constituency he needed to implement housing reform.

Griscom's consciousness of this dilemma is evident in how he built his appeals for sanitary reform. Taking up the utilitarian perspective of the business community, he underscored the unique status of housing as a form of property that could and should be regulated without undermining fundamental rights of private property or contracts. Decent housing, he suggested, was itself necessary to preserve the value of other commodities, particularly the commodity of labor power. Inadequate housing would undermine the growth of the city's economy by producing a chronically sick and unstable work force, he warned, and unless housing were regulated, taxpayers would bear new expenses when the residents of tenant houses were "thrown upon public charity for support by the premature death or illness of heads of families." Griscom even went so far as to cost out the loss to the city of the value of 268 laborers' premature deaths ($44,616 a year over a twenty-year period). Only by seeing the cash value of workers' lives and health, he implied, could propertied New Yorkers be moved to take action.[26]

Although he verged on examining some of the underlying social relations that concentrated laboring families in crowded domestic quarters, when it came to positive remedies Griscom turned back to the physical solutions of forbidding nuisances, improving utilities, and altering design. Recognizing that builders would not produce affordable, healthy housing for the city's working people unless it was profitable, he, like other housing and health reformers, thought that "benevolent capitalists" must demonstrate through philanthropy alternative ways to build and manage healthy multifamily housing while still maintaining a "fair" return on their investment. His suggestion for the philanthropy of building tenements was taken up by the press. Appealing to the "law of Christian charity," the Whig *Morning Courier and Enquirer* suggested to its readers that property owners had a "duty" to provide "good, whole and healthy dwellings for the poor." "Twenty or even more poor families might well be accommodated in a single tenant house erected for that special purpose," it went on to explain, "and such houses built entirely for comfort without respect for show . . . could be erected at a very cheap rate and would command a rent sufficiently increased to cover any falling off of profits."[27] By this logic, any builder who erected a tenement could claim a benevolent fulfillment of duty, but few laboring families could afford to pay for the "philanthropy" of sufficiently increased rents.

The model tenement movement gained strength at the very moment that the production of purpose-built tenements was emerging as a new field of real estate investment. Three decades of concentrating working-class rents through subdivision had demonstrated to builders and landlords alike the profitability of purpose-built multifamily dwellings, particularly when they were erected without the "amenities" of light and air or plumbing. And few builders saw why *they* should be held to laws of Christian charity so readily transgressed by the propertied citizens in all other fields of investment and exchange.

Sanitary reformers stressed that a better design for multifamily dwellings could in and of itself solve the now linked housing and health crises, but a fine line existed between vernacular and "model" tenements. Low wages and chronic unemployment meant that wage-earning families would share apartments in new as well as old buildings. By the 1850s, tenements had become the dominant form of working-class housing and the number of cellar dwellings began to decline, but taller buildings with multiple apartments only gave landlords more space to subdivide and wage-earning tenants more space to share. In the 1840s, city inspectors and reformers in the Association for Improving the Condition of the Poor had hailed "recently built tenant houses" as the "best habitations for the laboring classes." "From so promising a beginning, much that would be advantageous was expected," reformers observed in 1853. "But after a time an unlooked for deterioration in the character of the buildings was manifested. Many were erected on so contracted and pernicious a scale as to be inferior, as it respects the essentials of a dwelling, to the old buildings whose place they were intended to supply."[28]

In the years 1845 to 1854, the citywide mortality rate reached its all-time high (40 deaths per 1,000 city residents), and the gap between death rates in middle-class and working-class districts widened dramatically. Because this decade of economic recovery and increased immigration followed on the heels of the 1837–1844 depression, the supply of working-class housing— whether in subdivided older buildings or in the new tenements now being constructed—fell far behind the need and well below the housing standards of an earlier generation of wage-earning families. More than two-thirds of the people who died annually in New York were children; by the early 1860s, children of immigrant parents were ten times more likely to die by the age of twenty than were the children of native-born parents.[29]

Early death was not the greatest danger that propertied New Yorkers saw in working-class housing conditions, however. In the 1850s, trade unionists and land reformers in the Industrial Congress began to elaborate a critique of capitalist social relations, including the wage relation. This collective organizing threatened to transform the terms of discussion of the condition of the laboring classes from greedy landlords and victimized tenants to questions of class powers in their largest sense. In this context, some editors and reformers began to read the housing crisis as a threat not only to health but also to social order. Tenement life constituted an "associated community" and "practical Fourierism," the *Courier* had warned, that would "destroy those feelings of attachment and of moral responsibility, which belong to the idea of the home."[30]

Public health reformers like Griscom assigned a priority to housing reform as the most effective safeguard of public health, morals, and order, but at some points Griscom's efforts to understand the workings of the housing market brought him into alliance with labor activists and land reformers. In 1853, for example, Griscom and his associate Robert Hartley (president of the Association for Improving the Condition of the Poor, which led the campaign for housing reform) rejected another panacea for health that had gained currency in sanitary reform circles abroad. English health reformers in the late 1830s campaigned to create new public walks and parks to serve as the "lungs" of industrial cities. Wealthy New York City merchants and uptown landowners, who in the early 1850s proposed the creation of Central Park, hoped to create a refined setting for their own socializing. But seeking to establish the *public* value of their project, they also invoked the language of English sanitary reformers and claimed that the park would improve the health and morals of the city's working people. Land reformers and members of the Industrial Congress denounced the park—not inaccurately—as a class-interested scheme of the "codfish aristocracy" and land speculators. And although their language was more tempered, Griscom and Hartley joined this protest. To remove more than seven hundred acres from the land market, they argued, would only introduce new pressures on the housing market and thereby increase rents and crowding. A park located more than three miles from the center of population, moreover, would afford little relief to congested working-class neighborhoods. If the city wished to serve public health by creating public lungs, Griscom suggested, it should build multiple small parks in working-class neighborhoods.[31]

In working-class circles, mid-nineteenth-century discussions of health and housing reform spilled over into a larger debate over how the city would come to terms with capitalist market relations. But sanitarians' focus on housing also offered wealthy and middle-class New Yorkers a way to contain that discussion by narrowing what topics could be addressed under the rubric of "public health." After Griscom's innovative term as city inspector, other city inspectors and reform groups predictably singled out the miserable conditions of tenant housing as the locus of disease, warned of the dangerous impact on the morals of the working class, and decried rapacious landlords. In 1853, the AICP conducted a ward-by-ward survey of housing conditions, a strategy taken up in 1856 by the first of a series of state senate and assembly investigative committees, and then by the Citizens' Association Council of Hygiene, which produced a systematic survey of housing conditions in 1865. Despite their sincere sympathy and intention of mobilizing a reform movement, these investigations also helped shape a new interpretation of social relations that in effect naturalized class divisions as a permanent feature of the city landscape. Presenting the city as irrevocably divided into "sunshine and shadow," the surveys—and journalists' similar investigations—drew a grim picture of victimization and continued to denounce greedy landlords; they also implied that there was no active relationship between the city's wealthy (and healthy) households and the conditions of the laboring population.[32]

The housing investigations, moreover, paved the way for the translation of relations between people into the statistical abstracts of social science. The reports presented a static picture of the effects of half a century of capitalist development. And in systematically documenting the numbers and density of tenements (which housed three-quarters of the city's families by 1866), reformers omitted information that might illuminate what caused thousands of New Yorkers to inhabit, as the Council of Hygiene described it in its 1865 report, "domiciles which invite and localize the most disabling and fatal kinds of disease." Instead of investigating what employers paid workers, the frequency and rate of unemployment, or the rate of capital accumulation in the city, the investigations drew a bleak and often sentimental portrait of demoralization that implied a different narrative of causation. Poor housing itself caused poverty by breeding indolence and despair alongside disease; left unattended, such housing would produce the dissatisfaction that fueled such extremes of class anger as the 1863 draft riot. Better housing would inspire the ambition, diligence, and discipline that allowed workers to help themselves and earn the means to enjoy the standard of living attained by the city's leading citizens. These surveys fueled the movement for developing building codes and sanitary inspection as a means of guaranteeing better housing, but they also erased from the discussion of health and housing conditions reflection on the larger system of economic relations that produced them.[33]

Griscom and his followers built a broad coalition in support of new housing and health regulations. Fire insurers, who had repeatedly and successfully pressed their own interests in regulating the built environment, now joined in the campaign for a building code that would reduce their risks further. Members of the new Republican party saw an opportunity to undermine the local power of Tammany Democrats by creating a state-appointed health board; physicians saw in such a body the enhancement of their authority as public experts. Merchants pursued their business interests in maintaining the city's reputation as a healthy and prosperous center of trade, and manufacturers subscribed to the theory that better housing would produce better-disciplined as well as healthier workers. The cholera epidemics of 1849 and 1865, and especially the 1863 draft riots, added urgency to reformers' campaign for new housing regulation, and in 1866 Radical Republicans in the state legislature heeded their calls by establishing the Metropolitan Health Board with new powers of sanitary inspection. The following year the legislature passed the city's first comprehensive housing act, which specified new construction standards—materials, room dimensions, provisions for light and air—as well as one toilet per twenty people.[34]

It says much for the effectiveness of Griscom and his followers that propertied New Yorkers would come to see the regulation of property rights in housing as in their interest. Yet the success lay not so much in establishing the principle that government could intervene in economic relations on behalf of a common good as in isolating housing as a special form of property. Reformers succeeded in extending the common law of nuisances to regulate land use and housing without jeopardizing the contractual relations of exchange. The creation of minimum housing standards came on the heels of the final deregulation of other markets (the inspection of food products, for example), and in the midst of a growing debate over workers' proposals to regulate the labor market by passing an eight-hour law. Housing had been successfully separated from these other arenas of contractual relations, however. Landlords and builders had never been a favored group in the city, and by mid-century their class power vis-à-vis other factions of capital had waned. If the burden of guaranteeing that workers would be adequately housed could be placed on the shoulders of builders and landlords, employers could maintain their own contractual power and freedom. Indeed, if the state took an interest in the quality of workers' housing, it might defuse workers' militancy in demanding higher wages or shorter hours. The terms of landlords' accountability, moreover, were limited; although new laws lifted some tenant liability for rent if a dwelling was "uninhabitable," landlords had no obligation to guarantee that the apartments they rented were safe for occupancy or to make repairs on a regular basis. To have required this degree of accountability would have subverted the principle of *caveat emptor* that ruled in all other arenas of commodity exchange. The law empowered inspectors, not tenants, to judge when housing conditions justified public action to compel landlords to correct them.[35]

The producers of housing saw little reason why they should surrender the right to profit while other capitalists were given free rein. Small builders, especially, protested the new construction codes, which raised the costs of producing tenements, narrowed the margin of profit in a highly risky enterprise, and threatened, they argued, to reduce the supply of housing and thus produce a worse outcome than even shoddy tenements. Yet the real estate industry as a whole was not necessarily opposed to regulations that would discipline competition within the construction industry by standardizing the product. From the perspective of many large landowners and speculators, codes would increase the level of investment in construction throughout the city and thus enhance land values, adding to the "unearned increment" produced by social progress. Similarly, the largest builders, whose middle-class flats and apartments already met the mandated minimum standards, felt little direct pressure from regulation, and they welcomed the upgrading of tenements whose otherwise unsanitary conditions might devalue their own projects in the same neighborhoods.[36]

Building codes may have helped make life safer and more comfortable for thousands of New Yorkers by increasing the number of apartments that had fire escapes and better ventilation, light, drainage, and plumbing, but initially these regulations did little to transform the living conditions or improve the health of New York's laboring families. The panic of 1873 and the depression that followed exacerbated the housing crisis, taking back the ground that the organized labor movement may have briefly won in the late 1860s. Not only did unemployed workers have less money for rent and landlords less money to pay for repairs, hundreds of builders declared bankruptcy. The Department of Buildings, moreover, worked through compromise, bribery, and deliberate oversight in issuing permits for *new* buildings; inspectors applied the codes unevenly, if at all, with respect to older tenements and subdivided tenant-houses. Enforcement encountered both jurisdictional and political problems. Health inspectors could demand the correction of the worst nuisances, but they seldom had the staff or time to insure that *owners*—if they could be identified—complied with their orders. Even after the passage of more stringent laws (culminating with the 1901 Housing Act) that required proprietors of older buildings to meet new minimal standards, the number of new tenements built to code paled against the legacy of the older buildings that remained in violation. More important, the laws had little impact on how and in what numbers or density tenants occupied buildings.[37]

More pleasant though building and health codes may have made New York in the last third of the nineteenth century, there is little evidence that these codes in and of themselves improved public health. The city's death rate declined unevenly after the Civil War, but historians attribute this trend, which began prior to the passage of reform legislation, as much to the city's increased investment in sewers and water lines as to new regulations. That is to say, the city increased the opportunity for builders and landlords to introduce plumbing and water, but before the end of the century a building did not need running water or flush toilets to be deemed fit for habitation.[38] Access to better housing continued to depend primarily on access to decent wages and steady employment.

Housing reform on behalf of public health carefully circumscribed the larger issues of regulating market relations, of introducing principles of accountability directly into the "laws" of supply and demand. Indeed, sanitarians and their supporters viewed housing reform as an alternative to class politics that might address such issues. Thus, the same citizens who embraced housing and health reform in the 1860s opposed workers' efforts to legislate an eight-hour day at wage rates established by trade unions. Indeed, after 1867, some reformers' interest in housing and health reform waned in proportion to their anxiety about the labor movement's own definition of the causes of their condition. Dorman Eaton, who had drafted the Health Act, for example, quickly shifted his attention from sanitary reform to attacking the "excesses of democracy" when public workers and the labor movement demanded the eight-hour day—in his mind, a "communistic scheme of lifting up the lower levels of life in this city to comfort." And by 1873, the AICP was arguing that if workers were "not well-fed, well-housed, and well-clothed, it is neither owing to providential allotment nor to the oppression of human laws, but to their indolence, improvidence, and vice. Hence, no power should interpose between them and the divinely-appointed penalties."[39] Where propertied New Yorkers had succeeded in shedding their own accountability for the conditions of the laboring classes, the discoveries of scientific medicine only reinforced the identification of disease with forces outside human and social relations. If workers' living conditions improved by the end of the nineteenth century, the explanation lay as much with the labor movement's determination to assert a collective right to health and comfort in the largest sense as with either housing reform or the discoveries of scientific medicine.

Public health reform has seldom pushed beyond the frame of enlightened self-interest to ask what the improved living standards of one group have to do with the poor standards of another. At most, the concept of a trickle-down or filter suggest that once those at the top secure the new levels of material well-being, that degree of well-being eventually becomes available to those at the bottom. The language of health—and fear of "contagion"—helped shape a perception of shared costs that constituted the public interest in regulating land use. But the relationship among households was defined as one of proximity, of shared utilities and vulnerabilities, not as one between people, between one group who could rob another group of health in order to make their own lives more comfortable.

It is difficult, of course, to think about health in such abstract terms. There remains a vast gap between most people's concepts of "public health" and the health of the people they know. On a fundamental level, many people continue to regard the health of family or friends, workmates and acquaintances, with a kind of fatalism that probably differs little from that of colonial New Yorkers. Whatever the advances of medical science, viruses, cancers, and other diseases remain providences beyond human control. And early death remains tragic and ultimately eludes accountability precisely because there is no compensation or retribution that restores the loss. Anger at personal suffering, alongside fear, can fuel demands for prevention as a collective responsibility. But collective action runs up against the difficulty of isolating "health" within the larger fabric of daily life and imagining it as a fundamental right of free persons.

Discussion of health as the product of social relations has not advanced much since the nineteenth century; indeed, the concept of "public health" remains tied to discussions of how much private individuals are willing or able to pay, although more in terms of insurance and taxes than in the purchase of healthy homes. Or health is taken to represent something individuals pay for through their behaviors. That health is not a common right of all New Yorkers—or of all Americans—is hardly an indictment of capitalist economy alone. But today, as in the nineteenth century, American shy away from questions of social accountability. Medical science's identification of the nonhuman agents of disease has worked to reinforce the idea that the destruction of health requires scrutiny, investigation, and regulation of "externalities" in the extreme case but not in the common case of everyday social relations that allow some people to live well because others live poorly and die young.

Notes

1. Edward Lubitz, "The Tenement Problem in New York City and the Movement for its Reform, 1856–1867" (Ph.D. diss., New York University, 1970), 50–52.

2. Ibid.; John Griscom, *The Sanitary Condition of the Laboring Population of New York with Suggestions for Its Improvement* (New York: Harper & Bros., 1845).

3. William Blackstone, *Commentaries on the Laws of England*, ed. William Casey Jones (1788; reprint, Baton Rouge: Claitor's Publishing Division, 1976), 2302, 2360. New Yorkers regarded Blackstone as authoritative on common law. It is perhaps noteworthy that his chapter on offenses against the public health moved so quickly to the category "public police and economy," treating laws against bigotry and vagrancy as well as "common nuisances."

4. The investigative reports are quoted in James Ford, *Slums and Housing, with Special Reference to New York City* (Cambridge: Harvard University Press, 1936), 1:60–62. On responses to yellow fever epidemics, see also John Duffy, *A History of Public Health in New York City, 1625–1866* (New York: Russell Sage Foundation, 1968), 101–121.

5. Blackstone, *Commentaries*, 1790.

6. Duffy, *History of Public Health, 1625–1866*, 176–228.

7. Hendrik Hartog, *Public Property and Private Power: The Corporation of the City of New York in American Law, 1730–1870* (Ithaca, N.Y.: Cornell University Press, 1983), 203; John Teaford, *Municipal Revolution in America: Origins of Modern Urban Government, 1650–1825* (Chicago: University of Chicago Press, 1975), 102–106, 109.

8. Morton Horwitz, *The Transformation of American Law, 1780–1860* (Cambridge: Harvard University Press, 1977), 160–211 (contract), 207–210 (employers' liability); on landlord-tenant law, Elizabeth Blackmar, *Manhattan for Rent, 1785–1850* (Ithaca, N.Y.: Cornell University Press, 1989), 219–220, 232–235; *Vanderbilt v.*

Persse, 3 Smith 428 (Court of Common Pleas, 1854), at 430 (quote). Lawrence Friedman, *A History of American Law* (1973; New York: Simon and Schuster, 1985), 299–304, notes that the law of torts remained undeveloped in the United States until the mid-nineteenth century; when it was applied to industrial work conditions, the fellow servant rule spared employers the charge of negligence for injuries caused by other workers. See also G. Edward White, *Tort Law in America: An Intellectual History* (New York: Oxford University Press, 1980), 50–55, 60–61.

9. Elizabeth D. Bleeker, July 26, 1799, July 30, August 1, 2, 8, 9, 1803, Diary, 1799–1806, Rare Books and Manuscripts Division, the New York Public Library, Astor, Lenox and Tilden Foundations; Ford, *Slums and Housing*, 1:74–75.

10. *Commercial Advertiser*, February 2, 1803; April 15, 1807.

11. Catharine Beecher, *A Treatise on Domestic Economy* (New York, 1841), chaps. 5–7, 25–26; Jeanne Boydston, *Home and Work: Housework, Wages and the Ideology of Labor in the Early Republic* (New York: Oxford University Press, 1990), 129–130.

12. Blackmar, *Manhattan for Rent*, 87–94, 100–105, 193–199.

13. Charles E. Rosenberg, "Pietism and the Origins of the American Public Health Movement," *Journal of the History of Medicine* 23 (1968): 16–35; Carol Smith Rosenberg, *Religion and the Rise of the American City* (Ithaca, N.Y.: Cornell University Press, 1971), 91–96, 166–174.

14. *Annual Report of the City Inspector*, 1834, cited in Ford, *Slums and Housing*, 96.

15. Board of Aldermen, *Documents*, 2, no. 36, 160.

16. Eugene Moehring, *Public Works and the Patterns of Urban Real Estate Growth in Manhattan, 1835–1894* (New York: Arno Press, 1981), chapters 2, 4.

17. William Gibbons to Charles Osborn, September 16, 1842, Charles F. Osborn Papers, Rare Books and Manuscripts Division, the New York Public Library, Astor, Lenox and Tilden Foundations.

18. See William Gibbons account in Charles F. Osborn and George L. Osborn, Account Books, Rare Books and Manuscripts Division, the New York Public Library, Astor, Lenox and Tilden Foundations.

19. Gibbons to Osborn, July 6, 1846, Osborn Papers.

20. Association for Improving the Condition of the Poor [hereafter AICP], *Fourteenth Annual Report* (1857), 25, quoted in Lubitz, "The Tenement Problem," 64.

21. Ford, *Slums and Housing*, 1:184–185. See also Roy Lubove, *The Progressives and the Slums: Tenement Housing Reform in New York City* (Pittsburgh: University of Pittsburgh Press, 1962), 92.

22. John Griscom, "Annual Report of the Interments of the City and County of New York for the Year 1842, with Remarks thereon and a Brief View of the Sanitary Condition of the City," Board of Assistant Aldermen, *Documents*, 9, no. 59, 160.

23. Griscom, "Annual Report . . . 1842," 156, 175.

24. Ibid., 175–176.

25. Griscom, *Sanitary Conditions*, 8–9; on subtenancy, see also Blackmar, *Manhattan for Rent*, 243–245.

26. Griscom, "Annual Report . . . 1842," 191–192, 203–204; Griscom, *Sanitary Conditions*, 42–48.

27. Griscom, "Annual Report . . . 1842," 176; *Morning Courier and New-York Enquirer*, January 13, 1847; see also January 28, 1847, and January 30, 1847.

28. AICP, *Tenth Annual Report* (1853), 26–27, New York Historical Society.

29. Duffy, *History of Public Health, 1625–1866*, 534–536.

30. *Morning Courier and New-York Enquirer*, January 30, 1847; on labor movement, Sean Wilentz, *Chants Democratic: New York City and the Rise of the American Working Class, 1788–1850* (New York: Oxford University Press, 1984), 363–390; Iver Bernstein, *The New York City Draft Riots: Their Significance for American Society and Politics in the Age of the Civil War* (New York: Oxford University Press, 1990), 75–124.

31. *New York Times*, June 30, 1853; Roy Rosenzweig and Elizabeth Blackman, *The Park and the People: A History of Central Park* (Ithaca, N.Y.: Cornell University Press, 1992), 24–25, 55.

32. For housing investigations, see Lubitz, "The Tenement Problem," 351–398, and, for example, "Report of the Special Committee on Tenements Houses in New York and Brooklyn," *Assembly Documents*, no. 199 (1856); "Report of the Select Committee Appointed to Examine into the Condition of Tenant Houses in New York and Brooklyn," *Assembly Documents*, no. 205 (1857); Citizens' Association of New York, *Report of the Council of Hygiene and Public Health* (New York, 1865); on the literary genre of a bifurcated city, see Peter Buckley, "To the Opera House: Culture and Society in New York City, 1820–1860" (Ph.D. diss., State University of New York at Stony Brook, 1984), 353–366.

33. Citizens' Association, *Report of the Council*, xv–xviii; Bernstein, *New York City Draft Riots*, 187, 188.

34. On housing and health reform coalitions and legislation, see James C. Mohr, *The Radical Republicans and Reform in New York During Reconstruction* (Ithaca: Cornell University Press, 1973), 32–34, 69–106, 139–152; Lubitz, "The Tenement Problem," 511–518; Duffy, *A History of Public Health, 1625–1866*, 540–570.

35. Blackmar, *Manhattan for Rent*, 235–236, 263–265.

36. Lubitz, "The Tenement Problem," 494–495.

37. On the subsequent history of housing reform legislation and failures of effective enforcement, see Roy Lubove, *The Progressives and the Slums: Tenement House Reforms in New York City, 1890–1917* (Pittsburgh: University of Pittsburgh Press, 1962), 28–32; Anthony Jackson, *A Place Called Home: A History of Low-Cost Housing in Manhattan* (Cambridge: MIT Press, 1976), 4–125.

38. For an evaluation of public health in New York in the second half of the nineteenth century, see John Duffy, *A History of Public Health in New York, 1866–1966* (New York: Russell Sage Foundation, 1974), 113–225, 619–621, and passim.

39. Dorman Eaton, Testimony in the Matter of Charges Against the Park Commission, December 7, 1876, box 81, file 24, Mayors' Papers, Municipal Archives and Record Center; AICP cited in Gordon Atkins, "Health, Housing, and Poverty in New York City, 1865–1898" (Ph.D. diss., Columbia University, 1947), 10.

Plagues and Prejudice: Nativism's Construction of Disease in Nineteenth- and Twentieth-Century New York City

On a mild April day in 1990, 65,000 angry marchers tied up lower Manhattan traffic after pouring across the Brooklyn Bridge, chanting and carrying placards protesting a new federal proposal on blood transfusions that stigmatized Haitians and Africans. The protesters—"college students, factory workers and families with picnic baskets and umbrellas to protect them from the sun"—were angered by a United States Food and Drug Administration recommendation that excluded all individuals from Haiti or the sub-Saharan region from donating blood on the grounds that these groups have large numbers of members who test positive for the HIV virus. The policy was not binding on blood banks, but because the FDA oversees the nation's blood supply, many local blood banks were complying.

Protesters contended that Haitians in the United States, who numbered 350,000 in the New York metropolitan area alone, were no more likely to carry the AIDS virus than any other group. Dr. Jean Claude Compas, chairman of the Haitian Coalition on AIDS, angrily told reporters, "This policy is on the basis that Haitian blood is dirty, that it is all infected with HIV virus. The decision is based . . . on nationality, ethnicity." Some in the crowd interpreted the recommendation as racist, describing such policies as evidence that AIDS is a weapon of "white folks." Others were less concerned by the motive than by the effect. Thirty-seven-year-old Herve La Guerre told the *New York Times*, "They're putting us in a position that we're not going to be able to survive here because uneducated people will discriminate against us if they think we have AIDS."[1] Several days later the FDA retreated from its recommendation in response to advice from its Blood Products Advisory Committee.[2]

The FDA's clumsy attempt to curb donations of HIV-positive plasma to blood banks was reminiscent of the early 1980s, when the Centers for Disease Control (CDC) in Atlanta sent a tremor of trepidation throughout New York and other areas of Haitian concentration by announcing that Haitian newcomers had been classified in a special high-risk category for AIDS. By 1985, when the CDC finally dropped Haitians from its high-risk list, the psychological, financial, and social damage had been done. Tens of thousands of Haitians in the United States and in Haiti, most not infected with AIDS, had lost jobs, housing, and educational opportunities.[3]

What did AIDS have to do with Haitian nationality? Apparently very little.[4] In April 1985, Dr. Walter Dowdle, director of the Center for Infectious Disease, acknowledged the spurious relationship, admitting, "The Haitians were the only risk group that were identified because of who they were rather than what they did."[5] Less than a decade later the Food and Drug Administration had only repeated the CDC's insensitivity.

The Haitians' plight was not unique among immigrants to America. Almost seventy years earlier, during the 1916 polio epidemic that crippled thousands of New Yorkers, visiting nurse Ida May Shlevin blamed foreign customs for the infection of three-year-old Jeanette, the daughter of Italian immigrants. Jeanette had been taken upstairs in the Brooklyn tenement by her parents to see the lifeless body of her friend, little Frances Lucianna, who had just become polio's latest victim. Jeanette had gently kissed Frances goodbye, and now the child was ill. Nurse Shlevin scoffed, "This [kissing the dead] seems to be a religious habit among the Italians."[6] In 1916, Italian immigrants in New York and other East Coast cities were feared as carriers of polio much as Haitians were later shunned as the bearers of AIDS.[7]

Americans have often welcomed newcomers contingent on their physical health and intellectual vitality, expressing a strong desire to admit only the most fit and able to the privilege of competing for the economic and social rewards of life in the United States. On other occasions the native-born have been equally emphatic in their confidence that their country's unique blend of individual liberty, capitalism, and political democracy could transform downtrodden and oppressed humanity from every corner of the globe into new and improved men and women, denizens of a country singled out by the Creator for special blessing. Always, Americans have believed that immigrants posed a threat. The debilities of the unfit might make them a burden rather than an asset to their new country; might spread infectious diseases among the native-born and shatter the well-being of the very society that offered newcomers freedom and opportunity.

In the United States, as in all other countries of the world, quarantine was long the first line of defense against illness from abroad. After the American Revolution, in 1784, New York's colonial quarantine laws were reenacted as state laws. Bedloe's Island in New York Harbor was the quarantine station; a port physician was in charge. He was responsible for inspecting all incoming vessels that he suspected of carrying infection and for reporting conditions aboard to the governor or the mayor, who would then decide whether a ship should be quarantined and for how long. Immigrants detained for any length of time were generally sent to the Marine Hospital at Red Hook.[8]

Because shipmasters sought to maximize profits by cramming into their holds as many immigrants as possible, shipboard illness and mortality was quite common. Typhus and diarrhea ravaged tightly packed passengers to the New World. Friedrich Kapp, one of New York's commissioners of emigration, recalled in 1870 that earlier in the century, "Ten deaths among one hundred passengers was nothing extraordinary; twenty per cent was not unheard of; and there were cases of 400 out of 1,200 passengers being buried before ships left port [in Europe]."[9] In New York, the Marine Hospital filled to capacity when several ships docked at the same time.

In addition to quarantine, medical inspection and exclusion of individual newcomers was undertaken as a further preventive measure to ensure the American public's health. Between 1840 and 1860, approximately 4.5 million immigrants arrived in the United States, mostly from Ireland, the German states, and other countries of northern and western Europe, with a noticeable migration from China, as well. Certification of these newcomers' health was a state matter. Because New York was the busiest portal to America, a disproportionate burden fell upon New York State officials. Over 2.3 million, mostly Irish and Germans, crowded into the port of New York alone.[10]

As early as the 1830s, Irish immigrants who lived in rundown shanties and tenements along New York's rivers were being blamed for importing the cholera epidemic (from which they suffered disproportionately).[11] Fear of cholera, especially after the epidemic of 1832, stimulated public demand for inspection of emigrants prior to departure. Soon, those who left from western European ports began to receive an exam from a physician employed by the country of departure, lest shiploads of emigrants be annihilated by cholera during the voyage.

A physician who made the crossing many times on American ships wrote a letter to the *New York Times* in 1851 describing an exam that bordered on charade. Each passenger "inspected" by the doctors was required to stick out his or her tongue, while the overburdened physicians barely glanced up from their papers.[12] Passengers infested with vermin, filth, or the early stages of smallpox were often overlooked. On busy days when several ships were departing, as many as a thousand travelers might pass before a team of two doctors who, standing behind a small window, asked each emigrant whether they were well, glanced at tongues through the glass partition, and stamped tickets speedily. American authorities did complain to British emigration commissioners, but their protests were dismissed. The British denied that they were casting sick emigrants upon the world's waters, arguing that most shipboard diseases were the result of changes in diet, seasickness, apprehension, and other physical and emotional conditions that compromised passengers' health, making them susceptible to disease only after departure.[13]

Medical inspections of emigrants were hardly thorough, but neither were they egregiously superficial, given the state of the medical arts. Mid-century medical knowledge, especially pertaining to infectious diseases, remained thin. Diagnostic techniques were primitive, and acute observation and experienced judgment were still the most reliable instruments.[14]

SCREENING NEW ARRIVALS

In New York, at the other end of the rigorous trans-Atlantic journey for most mid-century European emigrants, the inspection was equally casual. Beginning in the summer of 1847, however, the arrival of thousands of sick Irish immigrants in flight from famine compelled adoption of more systematic procedures.

In May 1855, Castle Garden, an old fort at the tip of Manhattan, was leased; after being renovated, it reopened on August 1 as an immigration reception center: New York's Emigration Landing Depot. It was the site for a medical inspection designed to exclude infectious disease from the port of New York. Vessels laden with prospective immigrants anchored at the Quarantine Station, six miles below New York City. There, a New York State emigration officer boarded to count passengers and record midpassage deaths, as well as the degree and kind of illnesses that passengers had suffered during the journey. A report was sent to the general agent and superintendent at Castle Garden.

Passengers were then taken to Castle Garden for an individual medical inspection. After the examination, migrants were directed into a rotunda in the center of the depot, where they registered their names, nationalities, former places of residence, and intended destination. Thus, by the mid-1850s, every newcomer was subjected to two medical examinations—one upon departure and the other upon landing—and the more general inquiry of the quarantine officer.[15]

Clearly, disease prevention by inspection was on the minds of state and local officials in New York. Not until the last decade of the nineteenth century, however, did the federal government join in efforts to bar the door against immigrants who might pose a public health threat. Periodic cholera epidemics, broad acceptance of the germ theory of disease, and millions of newcomers spurred Congress to give federal authorities responsibility for protecting public health from infectious diseases.

Between 1880 and 1924, 23.5 million immigrants arrived in the United States, largely from countries in southern and eastern Europe, but also in smaller numbers from China, Japan, Mexico, and Canada. Federal immigration depots were built and administered with the intent of protecting the natives from the newcomers. Because New York was the busiest port of entry for immigrants, the Ellis Island depot was opened in 1892 as the flagship immigration station. In 1907, the peak year for immigration in the twentieth century, 1,285,000 immigrants entered the country; 866,660 (67.4 percent) were processed on Ellis. By the time the Ellis Island depot finally closed in 1954, 12,000,000 newcomers had entered the United States through its doors. Physicians charged with examining the first arrivals on Ellis Island were already converts to the germ theory of infectious disease that emerged from the research of Robert Koch in Germany. Five years earlier, the federal government had ordered the beginning of cholera studies, albeit with limited facilities. In one room on the ground floor of the Marine Hospital at Stapleton, Staten Island, Dr. Joseph Kinyoun fought the opening rounds of the federal govrnment's battle with bacteria—in this case, the germs responsible for Asiatic cholera. That war for the nation's health soon escalated. It fell to the physicians of the United States Marine Hospital Service, renamed the United States Public Health Service (PHS) in 1912, to serve on the nation's borders as medical sentries responsible for preventing the invasion of harmful bacteria from abroad.[16]

Ships entering New York's harbor after 1890 first passed quarantine, which was still supervised by New York State public health inspectors. These guardians of the public's health boarded arriving ships searching for cases of typhus, cholera, plague, smallpox, or yellow fever—all major epidemic diseases. When state officers in charge of quarantine finished their interrogation of the ship's doctor and captain, they left. Then came physicians from the PHS boarding division, who perfunctorily inspected in their cabins well-off passengers who could afford first- or second-class accommodations. Class biases of the era and pressure from steamship companies anxious to avoid inconveniencing wealthy clientele abbreviated the hunt for disease among the affluent. Only newcomers traveling third class and steerage were ferried to Ellis Island to stand the line inspection conducted by PHS physicians.

As they climbed the stairs to Ellis's main hall, immigrants lugging their hand baggage were already being scrutinized by PHS physicians for signs of abnormal physical stress that might signal more than fatigue after a long journey. Hearts could be assessed as strong or weak following the climb, and the physical stress would reveal clues to illnesses or malformations. The stairs were the first hurdle in the line inspection, an orderly procedure developed by the PHS to inspect efficiently large numbers of immigrants with limited numbers of doctors.

Of special concern to immigration and public health officials were highly contagious diseases such as trachoma and favus. Trachoma was an eye infection and favus a scalp disease. In 1898, the examination for trachoma was given only to those who exhibited readily visible symptoms or who seemed to be suspiciously trying to hide their eyes. Beginning in 1905, however, federal physicians at immigration depots everted all immigrants' eyelids. Because no specialized instrument yet existed, physicians used slender metal button hooks more commonly used to assist ladies in fastening their long, fashionable gloves or high-button shoes. The doctors sterilized their instruments between examinations with a quick dip of the hook into a solution or a wipe on a Lysol-impregnated towel. Another doctor probed newcomers' scalps for evidence of favus fungi.

In fiscal 1911, a fairly typical year during the 1890–1924 peak period, 749,642 aliens were examined by the PHS; 16,910 of them were certified for physical or mental defects. Of these, 1,363 had loathsome or dangerous contagious diseases. The number of immigrants returned to their ports of origin never exceeded 3 percent of the new arrivals in any given year, and the average for the entire period was well below 1 percent. Medical inspection at American immigration ports, including Ellis Island, did not markedly reduce immigration to the United States. Rather, there was a sharp increase in the percentage rejected for medical instead of economic or political reasons. From less than 2 percent in 1898, it increased to 57 percent in 1913 and 69 percent by 1916.[17]

In part, the increase in medical exclusions was due to improved diagnostic techniques, especially important in detecting diseases less visibly apparent than trachoma and favus. One of the most feared diseases of the nineteenth and early twentieth centuries was tuberculosis. In 1891, when PHS doctors first began their examination routine, tuberculosis was generally diagnosed by auscultation, using a stethoscope to listen for the sounds that cavities in diseased lung tissue produced.[18] By 1910, taking chest X-rays was common practice, as were laboratory analyses of residue from patients' lungs. Still, even with improved technique many of those infected with TB abroad slipped through. A slide showing the tubercle bacillus in an immigrant's sputum was the sole sufficient evidence to bar a newcomer with TB, and not every newcomer was tested.[19] In general, only those whose bodies were wracked with active TB were intercepted on Ellis. The 315 newcomers rejected for TB in 1918 (2.3 percent of those certified for rejection on medical grounds) were the most in a single year during the entire peak period. Prevention through inspection had its limitations.

THE 1916 POLIO EPIDEMIC

Long a mecca for immigrants after their arrival, New York City is a laboratory for exploring the relationship of infectious disease to prejudice against the foreign-born who managed to enter the "golden door." The 1916 polio epidemic suggests how immigrants, and often a specific nationality, were stigmatized by association with a particular disease. Armed with the latest public health regulations and the power to enforce them, municipal officials sought to deflect prejudice with truth and preventive measures. Still, some immigrants found themselves the victims of an epidemic of intolerance every bit as virulent as the crippling virus gripping the city.

Polio epidemics in western Europe and the United States were rare prior to

1907, when a major epidemic hit New York and killed an estimated 2,500 persons.[20] After 1907, polio deaths rose considerably; between 1910 and 1914 approximately 30,000 cases were reported across the country, including 5,000 deaths from the disease. Ironically, the very improvements in personal hygiene and public sanitation that were eliminating epidemics of typhoid and cholera contributed to the fresh virulence of polio. We now know that polio viruses previously infected most infants and young children and generally produced immunities rather than devastating illness. However, as improved sanitation killed off the milder, immunity-giving viruses, it made young victims more vulnerable to more potent, crippling viral strains. In the summers of 1907 and 1910, young New Yorkers from affluent and poor families alike were felled in large numbers.[21]

Each summer, New York health authorities stood watch. In 1916, even as the world's attention was turned to the war that was devastating Europe, polio again attacked New York City's children. The first case was reported on June 6 from a heavily populated section in Brooklyn, near the waterfront. Visiting nurses were ordered to make a search of nearby tenements, and, apartment by apartment, they pinpointed another twenty-two victims. Some had been stricken with illness for several weeks but their families had not called in a physician. Many were Italian immigrants.

By 1916, millions of Italian immigrants, most from the south of Italy, had arrived in the United States. Many settled in the New York area, at least initially. In New York, the polio death rate per 1,000 estimated population of children under ten years of age was 1.63 for Italian children, well below the 3.42 for the native-born or the 3.27 for German youngsters. The reasons remain unknown, but as Health Commissioner Haven Emerson observed, "Certainly the social and economic conditions under which these people live are no more favorable than those under which the Americans, Germans, and Irish live, among whom the mortality of the disease is the highest."[22] The 1,348 polio cases contracted by those of Italian nativity in New York City was the highest for any immigrant group, however, second only to the 3,825 cases among the native-born.[23]

By their very nature epidemics are intense, and polio epidemics struck suddenly, in summer, when youngsters were enjoying the freedoms of childhood.[24] Because there were so many Italian immigrants and because they lived in tightly concentrated neighborhoods, and because immigrants were viewed by many as a marginal and potentially subversive influence upon society, the incidences of Italian polio made a disproportionate impact on the imagination of a public already shaken by the virulence of the epidemic and the youth of many victims. Were the victims being blamed for the disease?

The newly elected mayor, John P. Mitchel, and his very capable health commissioner, Dr. Haven Emerson, were not bigots, but neither did they understand the origins of polio or how it was spread. Its appearance among the

Italians prompted formal inquiry into whether the epidemic had been imported. On July 1, 1916, the *New York Times* reported that Emerson had heard rumors that the Italians were responsible for the epidemic.[25] Hoping to either confirm or quell the story, Dr. Emerson contacted the quarantine station in the lower part of New York Bay. Quarantine officers reported that no newcomers with the disease had been detected and that there was no word from Italy regarding epidemics there.[26]

Next Emerson turned to Washington. Through officials on Ellis Island, Emerson inquired of PHS Surgeon General Rupert Blue whether the service had detected any Italians headed for Brooklyn after May 15, 1916. He also asked Blue whether American consular officials abroad were reporting "the prevalence of poliomyelitis" in Italian ports, especially "Genoa and Naples," from which America-bound ships had recently disembarked.[27]

In a memorandum to Blue, PHS surgeon C. H. Lavinder made it clear that he found Haven Emerson's inquiry reasonable for several reasons. First, early cases had been concentrated "among Italians of the Immigrant class in Brooklyn." Second, there were rumors that "infantile paralysis has recently been prevailing extensively in the Italian maritime cities from which comes Italian immigration." Third, the marked difference in the clinical type of the disease from earlier epidemics and the "greatly increased virulence of the infection" suggested "the importation of a new strain of the virus."[28] No cases appeared in Ellis Island hospital records, however. Certainly, the two-week journey and the detention of a certain percentage of every shipload would have revealed at least a few cases among the detained if Italy were the source of the problem. Just to be thorough, Italian officials were queried through the American consul. There were no epidemics of infantile paralysis in ports of disembarkation.[29]

The Italian connection was not simply discredited and abandoned by municipal officials. What link did they see between immigrants and polio? The answer appears to be filth, especially filth resulting from the sanitary habits and personal hygiene of newcomers. Even as they searched for the living organisms responsible for infantile paralysis, public health professionals could not completely wean themselves from sanitarian patterns of thought. Words and deeds often clashed with germ theory in the absence of certainty about how one contracted polio. Although there were ample cases of polio among children of the native-born middle class, those desperate for answers continued to stigmatize vulnerable newcomers.

The Italians, mostly impoverished workers from the southern provinces, were frequently denigrated by critics for unsanitary living conditions. In 1890, Richmond Mayo-Smith, a Columbia University professor of political economy, described Italian immigrants in New York's tenements: "Huddled together in miserable apartments in filth and rags, without the slightest regard to decency or health, they present a picture of squalid existence degrading to any civilization and a menace to the health of the whole community." Italians, heirs to one of the world's oldest civilizations, seemed to Mayo-Smith to be "ignorant, criminal and vicious, eating food that we would give to dogs." Their "very stolidity and patience under such conditions show that they lack the faintest appreciation of what civilization means," he added.[30]

Nor was the association of Italians and polio in New York State completely unprecedented. During the 1910 polio epidemic, an occasional report made the connection between group and disease, though the precise nature of that linkage was vague. In the upstate New York community of Eldridge, Dr. Milton Gregg recorded in his case notes on polio victim Mary Hill that "an Italian road construction gang in the neighborhood" was quite likely responsible for the disease's outbreak.[31]

In the summer of 1916, during the height of the epidemic, New York public health officials turned to education and even stronger preventive action to curb polio where many thought it was originating—among the immigrants. Italian neighborhoods were deluged with health department pamphlets and signs in the Italian language warning immigrant mothers about polio and urging them to be hygienic in their personal habits and child-rearing practices. The Department of Social Betterment of the Brooklyn Bureau of Charities issued 100,000 leaflets printed in Italian, Yiddish, and English.[32] Although all public gatherings of the urban poor, including block parties and public playgrounds, were sometimes monitored by health officials, the Italians were frequently singled out. In New York City, the three-day *festa* of our Lady of Mount Carmel was canceled by order of the Health Department.[33] Although Eastern European Jews and Polish immigrants were sometimes also mentioned as carriers of polio, Italians were assigned most of the blame.

Thomas J. Riley, general secretary of the Brooklyn Bureau of Charities, toured the neighborhood where the epidemic was most intense, using a map "showing by red dots every ill-fated house or tenement." He also went armed with reason. On the relationship of the neighborhood to the disease he wrote, "The reasonable thing to say is that dirt does not cause infantile paralysis or cause the germ to multiply, but that in all probability, it does help to spread the infection." The sympathetic Riley did not blame Italians as a group for the epidemic. Instead, he hoped that "good municipal housekeeping" would eventually help to "bring the humblest family in our midst a fair chance for a wholesome living." In the meantime, he could only hope for "something more heroic than treating the symptoms."[34]

When education and bans on public assembly proved insufficient, quarantine was tried. The decision to quarantine a household was made upon the recommendation of visiting nurses. Public health nurses who climbed tall tenement staircases to report on polio cases as part of New York City's Special Investigation of Infantile Paralysis under the Rockefeller Institute's Dr. Simon Flexner were often angry and impatient with Italian families. Not surprisingly, nurses possessing the power to recommend that a family be confined to its home were often feared and resented as intruders by Italian immigrants, especially the parents of children stricken with the disease. To these newcomers disease often was a manifestation of a stranger's ill will, and cures could only arise from prayers answered by divine intervention.[35] Mutual distrust, then, nourished an anti-Italian sentiment in many of the nurses' reports. After visiting one-year-old Petro Pollizzi, one nurse wrote, "These people neither understand nor speak Eng. [sic] so I could get very little accurate information. . . . These people are very ignorant and suspicious."[36] Often the nurses noted whether families with stricken children were being treated by an Italian physician, with the implication that the care of such doctors was suspect.

Members of the Italian community did not hesitate to publicly deny the relationship between ethnicity and polio and to point properly to anti-Italian nativism as the source of the stigma. One writer who refused to give his last name wrote to Mayor Mitchel, denouncing the prejudice. He fumed, "I wish to say emphatically that the American Italian is not to be singled out and charged with anything." Italians' only culpability was "nationality," he wrote. The protester urged the mayor to consider poor sewage systems and inadequate garbage disposal facilities as the source of the scourge.[37]

More often, though, impoverished and fearful Italian immigrants simply resisted what they perceived to be the intrusion of health officials who might even be spreading the disease themselves simply by going from house to house. Apprehensive immigrant parents often barred their doors to visiting nurses. On at least one occasion, those who traditionally offered "protection" to Sicilians brought Old World patterns of intimidation to the new. A pediatric clinic nurse who often reported cases of polio and violations of the sanitary code in a Brooklyn neighborhood known as Pigtown had her life threatened in a letter sent by the "Black Hand," or Mafia. After that she was escorted to and from the clinic by a policeman.[38]

Most Italian immigrants did not turn to the Black Hand to protect them from visiting nurses, and many physicians and public health officials well understood that the Italians were unconnected to the polio epidemic except by being among its victims. When the polio epidemic ended by itself with the first frosts of October 1916, the fraudulence of the charges against the Italians and the inadequacy of medical science to curb polio were equally apparent.

RESPONSES TO PREJUDICE AND DISEASE

Even as individual families dealt with being stigmatized by firing off indignant letters and slamming their doors in the face of municipal health workers, ethnic groups were developing broader, more coordinated responses in defense of newcomers burdened by the twin plagues of disease and prejudice.

Eastern European Jews were often associated in the public mind with tuberculosis, or consumption as the disease was often called. "It came to be re-garded as 'a Jewish disease,' or 'the tailors' disease,'" according to historian Irving Howe, because so many young Jewish consumptives earned their liv-ings with a needle.[39] Tuberculosis was neither peculiar to Jews nor to those who worked in the garment industry, yet Jews were stigmatized as carriers of tuberculosis. In part, the emaciated appearance of consumptives was equated with the feeble appearance and behavior that many nativists attributed to Jew-ish arrivals. Nativist scholar E. A. Ross at the University of Wisconsin espe-cially worried about the arrival of so many Jewish immigrants, over two million of whom would pour into the United States by the mid-1920s. To Ross's eye they appeared wasted and lacking in the physical vitality that he attributed to America's sturdier Anglo-Saxon stock. In 1914 Ross wrote, "On the physical side the Hebrews are the polar opposite of our pioneer breed. Not only are they undersized and weak muscled, but they shun bodily activity and are exceedingly sensitive to pain." Physical descriptions of those suffering from consumption were often appropriated by Ross and others for their de-scription of Jews' physical appearance.[40]

The Jewish community mounted a dual response to smears aimed at the health and vitality of the group, especially those barbs pertaining to tuber-culosis. Jewish health experts collected, analyzed, and published data that not only refuted the notion that Jews were especially prone to tuberculosis, but in fact suggested that rates of consumption among Jews both in Europe and in the United States were lower than rates for non-Jews. In addition, Jewish philanthropists financed health care for the Jewish indigent and built hospitals and sanitariums that lifted the burden of health care from the communities with high concentrations of Eastern European Jews. The aim was to defuse charges that tubercular Jews were becoming public charges in their new country.

Throughout the nineteenth century and the first decades of the twentieth, consumption had become the foremost killer of humanity among infectious diseases. Once a diagnosis of consumption was confirmed it was universally held to be incurable. Striking especially those between the ages of fifteen and thirty-five, the most productive and otherwise healthy period of life, it attacked the rich and/or famous such as Chopin, Napoleon, and Thoreau; the poorest; and those in between. If less spectacular in its effects on large con-centrations of human population than epidemic diseases such as cholera and yellow fever, consumption was no less feared. Expressions of concern about consumption filled the popular press as well as professional journals. Because the disease was incurable, much of this literature aimed at identify-ing those individuals and groups who ran the most risk of developing con-sumption.[41]

Interestingly, even as Americans' concern increased, tuberculosis mortality rates were declining. Well before Robert Koch's 1880 discovery of the tubercle bacillus and the development of public health programs to control the disease's spread, mortality from tuberculosis began to decline among all segments of the population, beginning around 1840 in England and 1870 in the United States. Rates continued to decline until World War II, rose during the war, and then fell dramatically afterward, the result of antimicrobial treatment. The reasons are a matter of some historical controversy, but a persuasive case has been made that efforts to reduce the contact between those infected with pulmonary tuberculosis and those still uninfected dramatically shrank the opportunity for victims to spread their infection.[42]

At about the time that mortality from TB was beginning to decline, the TB mortality figures for Jews living in Europe were lower than for any other group. Tuberculosis was found less frequently among Jews residing in Russia, Austria-Hungary, and Rumania than among gentiles. For the years 1901–1903, for example, the distribution of pulmonary tuberculosis among various religious groups per 10,000 of the population in these countries were Catholics, 38.3 percent; Protestants, 24.6 percent; and Jews, 13.1 percent. For all forms of TB, the figures were Catholics 49.6; Protestants, 32.8; and Jews, 17.8. Death rates computed for various cities with high concentrations of Jews suggest a similar mortality pattern: Lemberg (the German name for Lvov), Jews, 30.64, Christians, 63.51; Cracow, Jews, 20.49, Christians, 66.41. But, as with Italians and polio, mere facts did not cloud the public mind in the association of Jews with tuberculosis.[43]

Dr. Maurice Fishberg, who served as medical examiner to the United Hebrew Charities in the late nineteenth century, provided a rare insight into the health of Jews residing in New York in that era. A physician and an immigrant himself, Fishberg had a special interest in tuberculosis that led him to serve as chief physician and director of the tuberculosis service of the Montefiore Hospital and later at other institutions, as well as to write a two-volume textbook, *Pulmonary Tuberculosis* (1916). His deep interest in anthropology led him into scientific investigation and data collection on all aspects of pathology among the Jews. Fishberg's data, and that of the other physicians cited in his studies, show that in wards inhabited mostly by Jews, the mortality rate from tuberculosis for the years 1897, 1898, and 1899 was less than that found in the twenty other wards of the city. The seventh, tenth, eleventh, and thirteenth wards, located on the Lower East Side and populated mostly by Jews, experienced mortality rates of 213.74, 172.44, 155.27, and 110.54 per 100,000 inhabitants respectively, while the fourth ward, which was populated largely by non-Jewish laborers, had a death rate of 565.06. An important correlate of TB is population density, and the figures become even more persuasive when we note that the average number of persons to the acre in the four wards on the Lower East Side was 487.7, compared with 146.4 in the other twenty wards of the city. Yet the average annual death rate from TB was 335.17 throughout the city compared to a low 162.9 for the Jewish wards.[44]

Fishberg was among those Jewish scholars determined to refute the notion of Jewish racial inferiority, a claim made perennially by anti-Semites to justify the ostracism and persecution of Jews.[45] He did not speculate about the possibility that certain genetic groups might have a greater or lesser propensity for immunity, a belief widely accepted today. Instead, while admitting that the evidence was hardly conclusive, Fishberg focused his attention on environment and culture in shaping Jewish characteristics, including patterns of health and disease.[46] He joined those who believed that the relatively high immunity of Jews to infection with TB had something to do with "the careful selection of carcasses in Jewish slaughterhouses" and the "infrequency of alcoholism and syphilis" among Jews.[47]

Whatever the reason for lower rates of TB among Jews than among other immigrant groups, socioeconomic class was a factor even among Jews. Data from Manhattan's fourth, sixth, eighth, and tenth assembly districts—mostly Jewish, immigrant poor—show TB rates of 11.9, 12.0, 13.5, and 11.7 per 1,000 persons, respectively. The thirty-first assembly district in Manhattan, consisting of wealthier Jews, shows a rate of merely 3.0 per 1,000. Even among the Jews, tuberculosis seemed to flourish most readily in the crowded, unhealthy conditions of the poorest sections of urban enclaves.[48]

Whether rich or poor, victims of tuberculosis faced extended treatment, no chance of full recovery, and a problematical chance of being able to resume a normal life after treatment. If diagnosed at what was considered an early stage, the disease sometimes responded to a change in climate and diet, although what climate and what diet differed from physician to physician. Preparations were prescribed to combat individual symptoms such as lung hemorrhage and cough, and opium was widely used to relieve the distress of the final stages.

THE SANITARIUM ERA

The closing decades of the nineteenth century witnessed the rise of sanitarium care. A German innovation, the sanitarium was introduced into the United States by New York physician Edward L. Trudeau in the 1870s after he was diagnosed as tubercular.[49] Sanitariums applied earlier therapies of beneficial climate, fresh air, and supervised nutritious diet to groups of patients in an institutional setting. The sanitarium could not offer a specific cure for tuberculosis, but it reflected a revision of the general view of tuberculosis from being incurable to being treatable. Various surgical techniques of collapsing seriously damaged lungs in the hopes of arresting the disease were also introduced at this time. It was not until after World War II, in 1947, that antibiotic therapy for TB began with the introduction of streptomycin and, later, even more effective drugs such as isoniazid. By 1960, once busy sanitariums would be abandoned or converted for use in fighting other diseases. However, in

1990 new cases of tuberculosis rose by more than 38 percent over the previous year in New York City, almost four times the rate of increase of 1989.[50] The trend has continued, making some public health professionals regret the absence of sanitariums to quarantine those with the disease and under treatment, thereby limiting its spread.[51]

The peak immigration period coincided with the era of sanitarium care for tuberculosis. Many thousands of poor immigrant workers stricken with TB were in need of costly extended care. Some expenses could be assumed by labor unions, mutual aid societies, or industrial insurance policies. Jewish *landsmannschaften*, mutual benevolent societies, provided benefits to members with TB, but most poor shop workers lacked sufficient coverage to defray the costs of a disease that drained individuals and organizations of health-care dollars even as it wasted the bodies of its victims. In response to the ubiquitous moan of Jewish consumptives, "Luft, gibt mir luft" (Air, give me air), Jewish physicians prescribed sanitarium care. One Jewish physician, knowing that some patients could not afford even a short sanitarium stay, prescribed rest and some cough medicine, writing on the prescription slip, "Join the Cloakmakers Union," presumably both to encourage unionism and to get the benefit of a sanitarium.[52]

Some sanitariums, such as Trudeau's facility at Saranac Lake, were located in upstate New York. Another, the Montefiore Sanitarium at Bedford Hills in Westchester County, was financed by Jewish philanthropists, especially the renowned financier Jacob Schiff and Lyman G. Bloomingdale, whose family founded the department store and who had himself lost a daughter to TB. The Montefiore Home for Chronic Invalids was opened in 1884, when the great wave of immigration to the United States was just beginning. Its supporters were philanthropists concerned by the plight of those for whom medicine offered little hope of a cure. The category included those with cancer, syphilis, the "opium habit," arthritis, chronic kidney disease, and chronic melancholy (what modern physicians might diagnose as clinical depression), and tuberculosis. A clean, warm place to rest, regular nursing, healthful food, and some assistance to relatives of the sick was all that could be done for incurables, but the expense for even that much was well beyond the means of poor Jewish immigrant laborers.[53]

The first Montefiore facility consisted of twenty-six beds in a small frame house on Manhattan's Upper East Side. Later facilities were located in Harlem and, later, in the northwest Bronx, then a green and healthful area on the fringe of the city. Doctors at Montefiore shared with others throughout the country the belief that fresh air, rest, good food, and regulated exercise made a successful regimen for treating patients in the early stages of TB. Disagreement was rampant over the details, however. What was more important—cold air or fresh air? What was the best climate and topography—the high altitude of mountains, or the low-lying desert?[54]

When the Montefiore trustees decided to build a separate tuberculosis sanitarium, they put their faith in altitude and opted for a site at Bedford, the "highest point in . . . [Westchester] county," which was also "entirely free from mosquitos and malaria," and only a forty-mile, ninety-minute railroad ride from New York City. Thus, patients could be transferred easily and physicians from home could come when needed "at slight cost to the institution."[55]

The Montefiore Sanitarium thrived as philanthropists such as the Lewisohn family contributed to the building of new pavilions, housing more beds. A 136-acre farm was also purchased. Farm work was part of the therapy for some of the patients, and the farm served as a source of food for all Montefiore facilities. Trustees hoped that the experience of country living might persuade some of those released to settle away from the congested urban tenements of New York where some might have contracted TB.

Many of the patients were only too aware of the conditions that had contributed to their illness and said so in patient publications. There were two literary societies—one conducted business in English and one in Yiddish, the language of recently arrived Eastern European Jews but disdainfully referred to as "jargon" by assimilated German Jewish physicians. Patient Bertha Pearl, who wrote in English for the *Montefiore Echo*, recounted a familiar immigrant experience in a 1916 article. "[You] sleep on the floor at our poor relation's. . . . Then your father dies, and your neighbors report you to the United Hebrew Charities, and you get less and less to eat till you get bananas and bread for a steady diet." It was conditions such as those remembered by Bertha Pearl that filled as many beds as Montefiore could assemble.[56]

When Montefiore found itself constantly filled, an increasing number of patients were recommended to other such facilities, especially those that shared the Montefiore doctors' confidence in the therapeutic powers of altitude. Facilities at Denver, Colorado, often received referrals from New York City.[57]

By the 1890s, Denver, with its clean, cold, dry climate, had already become a magnet for consumptives, many of them poor, Jewish, and from New York City.[58] Under the leadership of Rabbi William Friedman, a committee of Denverites pledged three thousand dollars and incorporated the Jewish Hospital Association of Denver to build a hospital for the care of respiratory diseases that, although built by Jews, would be open to all. Financial problems, some of them occasioned by the depression of 1893, slowed progress. However, when B'nai B'rith undertook to make the hospital a national institution for the care of tuberculosis patients, the National Jewish Hospital for Consumptives was truly on its way to becoming a reality. On December 10, 1899, the hospital opened, and, appropriately enough for an institution dedicated to serving all the suffering, the hospital's first patient was not even Jewish, but a twenty-five-year-old Swedish woman from Minnesota, Alberta Hansen.[59]

National Jewish opened with merely a sixty-five-bed capacity, but with only forty other TB sanitariums in the United States (and only five hundred beds in those devoted to treating TB patients), the new institution increased the number by 13 percent just by opening its doors. The combination of many applicants and too few spaces caused the institution to limit patient stays to six months and admit only those in the early stages of the disease, who had the best chance of some return to health. Formal application and a full medical exam were required of all applicants. All patients also had to show proof of having sufficient funds either to remain in Denver after discharge and be self-supporting or to return to their original home. The intent was to prevent National Jewish patients from becoming a burden to the larger Denver community and perhaps igniting an anti-Semitic backlash.[60]

National Jewish was founded for Jews by assimilationist German Jews, many of whom practiced Reform Judaism. Not all those that the institution hoped to serve were satisfied that the hospital was sufficiently sensitive to the spiritual needs of the growing number of Eastern European Jewish TB victims. Their religious practices were Orthodox and they needed care that combined medical therapy with opportunities for traditional religious observance. Unable to find a satisfactory synthesis of care and cultural climate at National Jewish, some of the newcomers turned to a new facility founded by others like themselves, the Jewish Consumptive Relief Society (JCRS).[61]

Twenty Eastern European Jewish tradesmen—a tinner, a furrier, a silk weaver, a tailor, a house painter, a cigar-maker, an actor, and a photographer among others—all victims of tuberculosis, met in October 1903 to found an institution that would meet their needs. It was a humble beginning. Among themselves, the twenty could raise only $1.10 for their Denver Charity for Consumptives.[62] After the name was changed to the Denver Appeal Society for Consumptives, to eliminate the word *charity* because of its condescending connotations, and an advertising campaign was launched in Yiddish and English, the idea gained some momentum.[63] Most of the contributions came from workers and their labor unions. A letter of February 28, 1908, thanked the Workman's Circle of New York for their contribution of $3.00.[64] A similar letter written several months later expressed appreciation to the president of the Rochester (New York) Workman's Circle for a personal donation of $1.35.[65] Agents of the JCRS combed Jewish communities around the country for donations, entreating philanthropists and placing *pushkes* (collection boxes) in stores, homes, and meeting halls for whatever coins a community could spare.[66]

The guiding light of JCRS was neither a rabbi nor a philanthropist. JCRS Secretary Dr. Charles Spivak was born Chaim Dovid Spivakofski in 1861 in Krementshug, Russia. A revolutionary socialist in his youth, Spivak was forced to flee Russia in 1882 to escape being apprehended by the secret police for his political activities. Arriving in New York at the age of twenty-one, Spivak held various jobs, from road paver on New York City's Fifth Avenue to millworker in Maine to farm laborer in New Jersey; eventually, he sought an education and a medical career. In 1890 he graduated from Jefferson Medical College in Philadelphia with honors, and by 1895 he was chief of staff of gastrointernal diseases at the Philadelphia Polyclinic. In 1896 his wife's poor health, very likely tuberculosis, caused the family to move to Denver, where Spivak continued to teach and practice at the University of Denver and Gross College of Medicine.[67]

Spivak's own immigrant background attracted him to the idea of a sanitarium that would offer care to those with traditional cultural and religious needs. The JCRS was formally dedicated on September 4, 1904; several days later six men and one woman became the society's first patients. They were housed in wooden tent cottages. Within a year, the patient population expanded to twenty and the number of tents increased to fifteen. Open to consumptives regardless of race or religion, as was National Jewish, the JCRS accepted those at all stages of the disease, at no charge. JCRS catered to the religious needs of those who practiced Orthodox Judaism, including careful observance of dietary restrictions.

German Jews and Eastern European Jews had long experienced cultural tensions in America. In the pages of the New York *Yiddishe Gazetten*, an Eastern European Jew contrasted the efficient charity of assimilated German Jews, with their "beautiful offices, desks, all decorated, but strict and angry faces," to *zedakah*, charity delivered with loving kindness as a religious obligation and experienced among his own Eastern European brethren "who speak his tongue, understand his thoughts and feel his heart."[68]

The cultural tensions that existed in New York City and elsewhere between German Jews and newer Eastern European arrivals were reflected in the relationship between National Jewish and the JCRS. Both sides gave as good as they got. Shortly after the JCRS was founded, it was attacked by National Jewish's Rabbi Friedman for extending "an open invitation to the Jewish communities of the United States to send their penniless consumptives to Colorado" and by bringing "incurable consumptives," posing a "dangerous menace to Colorado."[69] The JCRS defended its decision to accept cases of tuberculosis in advanced stages less on medical grounds than on humanitarian grounds, suggesting that the Jewish spirit of *rachmones* (mercy for the poor and suffering) was a higher standard than physicians' prognoses, which were derived from passionless medical science.[70] Rabbi Friedman countered that it was more humane not to raise false hopes in those with advanced cases by bringing them to Denver. Instead, he argued, it was "far better for the advanced consumptive to bear the ills he has, surrounded by family and friends, than to fly to greater suffering."[71]

In fact, both hospitals sought to combine care with a program of vocational training to avoid the possibility of turning loose an unemployable horde on Denver. National Jewish met its public responsibility with classes in English and a wide range of industrial classes. There were special classes in sewing and domestic sciences for women and even a national employment agent to assist ex-patients in finding jobs.[72] The JCRS, meanwhile, created shops to retrain workers in bookbinding, a trade that was "clean" and healthy for the lungs and offered immigrant Jews a niche in the marketplace. Even bookbinding could be controversial, however. The Colorado Board of Health wrote a letter to the JCRS, expressing concern over the handling, printing, and binding of books by consumptives. Somewhat reluctantly, the JCRS agreed to sterilize each book leaving the sanitarium and to affix a label to bookbindery products identifying them as having been made by patients.[73]

A thornier issue was the debate over the observance of the Jewish dietary laws of kashrut. This dispute cut to the heart of the differences between the highly assimilated German Jews who supported and administered National Jewish and the Eastern Europeans at JCRS. National Jewish did not observe the dietary laws because it was believed that tubercular patients needed a combination of milk, meat, and butter at all meals to restore their health. Dr. Moses Collins, an administrator at National Jewish, had maintained that following the Jewish dietary laws was "inadvisable for medical reasons."[74] For many Orthodox Jews, abandoning religious law was a step toward a fate worse than dying of consumption. The JCRS contended that patients need not abandon belief and tradition to recover their health. In an article entitled "Kosher Meat in Jewish Hospitals and Sanatoria," JCRS's Dr. Adolph Zederbaum argued that *kashrut* and better health were consistent. He wrote, "It is mere nonsense to claim that a sick person cannot thrive on Jewish meat and delicacies . . . at the Sanatorium of the JCRS dairy articles never appear together with meat." Moreover, he observed that by forcing patients to forsake dietary laws, more damage might be done to their health and general welfare than any positive nutritional value that might result by violating the laws.[75]

Denver had become an outpost of the New York Jewish community. Battles raging in Manhattan, Brooklyn, and the Bronx were transported west by the combatants. The conflict between competing tuberculosis sanitariums in Denver, each representing a different religious and cultural perspective within the Jewish community, is a reminder that illness not only precipitates struggles between natives and newcomers but also irritates existing tensions within ethnic groups over assimilation. Beyond that, it often widens the abyss between institutions and the individuals those institutions purport to serve.

THE PAST REFLECTED IN THE PRESENT

The peak of immigration to the United States occurred at the very time when modern scientific medicine was in its infancy. Twin fears of the stranger and the microbe triggered institutional responses both within the immigrant community and within the larger society, especially among those charged with overseeing the public's health. Times have changed, but as Susan Sontag and many others have observed, illnesses and values, lifestyles, even groups outside the American mainstream continue to be metaphors for each other and to fuel preexisting prejudices that underlay institutional reactions.[76]

In the early 1990s, the federal government continued to pursue institutional means of epidemic control to stop AIDS at the border, a means that stigmatizes immigrants of all nationalities. All applicants for immigration visas to the United States underwent mandatory blood testing and were excluded if they proved HIV-positive. As in earlier crises, the federal government had sought to use exclusion to control the epidemic; immigrants were subjected to mandatory testing for no clear epidemiological reason other than foreign birth. It was assumed that the stranger posed a health threat. Responses came from many quarters.

On September 9, 1990, Ellis Island, the largest historic restoration in American history, was reopened to the public. Guests waited in line for the boats that would ferry them to the ceremonies on the island, even as immigrants had waited for boats to ferry them in the opposite direction. Soon there was another reminder of Ellis Island's past. Those on line witnessed a demonstration by AIDS activists hoisting signs that protested HIV testing of immigrants and refugees and inadequate funding of AIDS research. One sign read, "Ellis Island 1892: opportunity—Ellis Island 1990: murder."[77] Hyperbole, of course. But also a demand that today's newcomers not be stigmatized as disease carriers who threaten to turn the United States into a colony of the world's diseased and dependent. The protesters' voices echoed the pain of yesterday's immigrants who feared lest their own bodies bar them from the opportunities that America promised.

Recent immigrant communities, too, mounted responses. In the early 1980s, Haitian spokespersons denounced the CDC's "high risk" categorization of Haitians as a national group. By the end of the decade, the call to end mandatory testing of immigrants went well beyond the Haitians, as did the march against the FDA's advice to refuse blood donations from Haitians and sub-Sahara Africans. And, as with earlier immigrants, voluntary organizations such as the Caribbean Women's Health Association, Inc., sought to promote prevention and care for their own. Community-produced videos shot in Haitian neighborhoods of Queens, New York, which dramatize the need to make sex safe from AIDS with condoms, were technologically innovative means to a familiar end.[78]

The faces and accents and diseases have changed in the great American debate over public health, but the underlying confrontation between native and newcomer remains constant. Because disease is socially and culturally constructed, plagues and prejudice are locked in a timeless embrace that merely grows tighter or looser from one era to the next.[79]

Notes

This article was written with the support of an Interpretive Research Grant from the National Endowment for the Humanities and is based in part on themes developed in Alan M. Kraut's book *Silent Travelers: Germs, Genes, and the "Immigrant Menace,"* published in 1994 by Basic Books, New York.

1. *New York Times*, April 21, 1990. See also *New York Post*, April 21, 1990.

2. Press release, "FDA Statement on the Blood Products Advisory Committee Recommendation," April 20, 1990.

3. The fullest discussion of the social and political controversy surrounding the Haitians and AIDS is in Paul Farmer, *AIDS and Accusation: Haiti and the Geography of Blame* (Berkeley: University of California Press, 1993). See also Dennis Altman, *AIDS in the Mind of America: The Social, Political, and Psychological Impact of a New Epidemic* (Garden City, N.Y.: Anchor Press/Doubleday, 1987), 70–74. The significance of the Haitian controversy to scientific efforts to identify the virus and its victims is in Randy Shilts, *And the Band Played On: Politics, People, and the AIDS Epidemic* (New York: St. Martin's Press, 1987).

4. Lawrence Altman, "Debate Grows on U.S. Listing of Haitians in AIDS Category," *New York Times*, July 31, 1983. Altman's article is also cited in D. Altman, *AIDS in the Mind of America*, 72.

5. Dr. Walter Dowdle as quoted in the *New York Times*, April 10, 1985.

6. Ida May Shlevin, Nurse, to Alvah. E. Doty, M.D., July 21, 1916, Nurse's Daily Report, Department of Health, City of New York, Special Investigation of Infantile Paralysis, B Category, Rockefeller Institute Papers, American Philosophical Society, Philadelphia, Pennsylvania. Kissing the dead is mentioned as part of the "ritualized outpouring of grief" in Rudolph J. Vecoli's "Cult and Occult in Italian-American Culture: The Persistence of a Religious Heritage," in *Immigrants and Religion in Urban America*, ed. Randall M. Miller and Thomas D. Marzik (Philadelphia: Temple University Press, 1977), 33.

7. Guenter Risse makes the analogy between the AIDS epidemic and the polio epidemic of 1916 in "Epidemics and History: Ecological Perspectives and Social Responses," in Elizabeth Fee and Daniel M. Fox, eds., *AIDS: The Burdens of History* (Berkeley: University of California Press, 1988), 48–56.

Saul Benison points to evidence that during the 1910 polio epidemic immigrants also had been blamed for the high incidence of the disease among their numbers. To demonstrate the ethnocentric social construction of the disease in some quarters, Benison cites a 1910 published letter to Dr. Simon Flexner of the Rockefeller Institute from a Mrs. A. O. Longmuir of Chouteau, Montana, who blames the appearance of polio on the "mode of living" of her Norwegian neighbors. She describes them as knowing "very little about sanitation or ventilation," noting that "under the kitchen floor they dig a cellar with neither light nor air" where they "keep bread, butter, meat, milk, and potatoes." To Mrs. Longmuir, "this alone would be a source of infection." As Benison observes, in a era before the disease was fully understood, the "seeming reasonableness" of this concerned woman's "analysis" was compelling to many contemporaries. See Saul Benison, "Poliomyelitis and the Rockefeller Institute: Social Effects and Institutional Response," *Journal of the History of Medicine and Allied Sciences* 29 (1974): 74–92.

8. John Duffy, *A History of Public Health in New York City, 1625–1866* (New York: Russell Sage Foundation, 1968), 86. The best volume on colonial immigration laws is Emberson Edward Proper, *Colonial Immigration Laws: A Study of the Regulation of Immigration by the English Colonies in America* (New York: AMS Press, 1967). The reaffirmation of many colonial laws in state legislation after independence is discussed most clearly in E. P. Hutchinson, *Legislative History of American Immigration Policy, 1798–1965* (Philadelphia: University of Pennsylvania Press, 1981), 388–404.

9. Friedrich Kapp, *Immigration and the Commissioners of Emigration* (1870; reprint, New York: Arno Press and the *New York Times*, 1969).

10. The best account of the era in New York is Robert Ernst, *Immigrant Life in New York City 1825–1863* (1949; reprint, Port Washington, N.Y.: Ira J. Friedman, 1965).

11. Charles Rosenberg, *The Cholera Years*, rev. ed. (Chicago: University of Chicago Press, 1987).

12. A letter from a "Doctor," *New York Times*, October 15, 1851.

13. The best study of the journey to America from Great Britain and Ireland during the mid-nineteenth century is Terry Coleman, *Going to America* (Garden City, N.Y.: Anchor Press/Doubleday, 1973).

14. By the mid-nineteenth century, the examination of the patient had progressed little beyond state-of-the-art medicine in the previous century. See Stanley Joel Reiser, *Medicine and the Reign of Technology* (New York: Cambridge University Press, 1978).

15. Kapp, *Immigration and the Commissioners of Emigration*, 105–124.

16. For a discussion of the medical examination on Ellis Island and how Progressives' "twin deities, science and bureaucratic efficiency, became the bulwark of the nation's defense of its physical health and social vitality" against the foreign born, see Alan M. Kraut, *Silent Travelers: Germs, Genes, and the "Immigrant Menace"* (New York: Basic Books, 1994), 50–77. Also, Elizabeth Yew, "Medical Inspection of the Immigrant at Ellis Island, 1891–1924," *Bulletin of the New York Academy of Medicine* 56 (June 1980): 488–510.

17. All percentages were calculated from data in U.S. Marine and Hospital Service [U.S. Public Health Service after 1912] *Annual Reports of the Surgeon General* (Washington, D.C.: Government Printing Office, 1892–1924).

18. Reiser, *Medicine and the Reign of Technology*, 29–30.

19. U.S. Public Health Service, *Regulations Governing the Medical Inspection of Aliens* (Washington, D.C.: Government Printing Office, 1917).

20. For a historical overview of the disease, see John R. Paul, *A History of Poliomyelitis* (New Haven: Yale University Press, 1971). For a discussion of polio epidemics in the United States prior to the 1930s, see Naomi Rogers, *Dirt and Disease: Polio before FDR* (New Brunswick, N.J.: Rutgers University Press, 1992), based on her dissertation, "Screen the Baby, Swat the Fly: Polio in the Northeastern United States, 1916" (Ph.D. diss., University of Pennsylvania, 1986). Also, Saul Benison, "The History of Polio Research in the United States: Appraisal and Lessons," in Gerald Holton, ed., *The Twentieth-Century Sciences: Studies in the Biography of Ideas* (New York: W. W. Norton, 1972), 308–343.

21. The 1916 epidemic in New York was chronicled by New York Health Commis-

sioner Haven Emerson, *A Monograph on the Epidemic of Poliomyelitis (Infantile Paralysis) in New York City in 1916 Based on the Official Reports of the Bureau of the Department of Health* (1917; reprint ed., New York: Arno Press, 1977). See also Emerson's presentation in "Transactions of a Special Conference of State and Territorial Health Officers with the United States Public Health Service, for the Consideration of the Prevention of the Spread of Poliomyelitis, Held at Washington, D.C., August 17 and 18, 1916," *Public Health Bulletin* 83 (1917); and C. H. Lavinder, A. W. Freeman, and W. H. Frost, "Epidemiological Studies of Poliomyelitis in New York City and the North-Eastern United States during 1916," *Public Health Bulletin* 91 (1918).

22. Emerson, *A Monograph on the Epidemic of Poliomyelitis*, 108–109.

23. Ibid.

24. Charles Rosenberg discusses the meaning of the epidemic as an event and its "dramaturgic form" in "What is an Epidemic? AIDS in Historical Perspective," *Daedalus* 118 (Spring 1989): 1–17.

25. *New York Times*, July 1, 1916.

26. *New York Times*, July 11, 1916.

27. Emerson's inquiry was documented in a cover letter and memorandum from C. H. Lavinder, the physician on Ellis Island who responded to the inquiry, to Surgeon General Rupert Blue in Washington, D.C., July 5, 1916, Record Group (RG) 90, File 1712, United States National Archives, Washington, D.C. (hereafter NA).

28. Ibid.

29. Memo from Acting Surgeon General to Eager at the American Consulate, Naples, Italy, July 6, 1916, RG 90, File 1712, NA.

30. Richmond Mayo-Smith, *Emigration and Immigration: A Study in Social Science* (New York, 1890), 133.

31. The Mary Hill case is cited in the papers of Dr. Simon Flexner at the American Philosophical Society in Philadelphia. See also Benison, "Poliomyelitis and the Rockefeller Institute," 81n19. Benison observes that immigrants were not the only minority groups blamed for spreading polio in 1910. He offers the example of Cotton Yates, a black farmer in St. Mary's County, Maryland, whose alleged responsibility for polio's spread made the Baltimore newspapers.

32. *New York Times*, July 9, 1916. Also, Rogers, *Dirt and Disease*, 47.

33. *New York Times*, July 12, 1916. Also, Rogers, "Screen the Baby, Swat the Fly," 39.

34. Thomas J. Riley, "Poverty and Poliomyelitis," *Survey*, July 29, 1916, 447–448.

35. Steeped in a culture centered on the domus and believing that illness resulted from a jealous stranger's *Mal'occhio* or "Evil Eye," Italians often preferred to seek health care from family members and cures from the intercession of holy figures, such as Harlem's Madonna of Mount Carmel, than from doctors and visiting nurses. See Robert Anthony Orsi, *The Madonna of 115th Street: Faith and Community in Italian Harlem, 1880–1950* (New Haven: Yale University Press, 1985). An earlier study aimed specifically at educating those who sought contact with the Italians community in the group's cherished folk culture is Phyllis H. Williams, *South Italian Folkways in Europe and America: A Handbook for Social Workers, Visiting Nurses, School Teachers, and Physicians* (New Haven: Yale University Press, 1938).

36. E. Holmes, Report of Nurse, August 24, 1916, Department of Health, City of New York, Special Investigation of Infantile Paralysis, A Category, Rockefeller Institute Papers, American Philosophical Society, Philadelphia, Pennsylvania.

37. Ernest J. C. to Mayor John P. Mitchel, July 10, 1916, Mayor John P. Mitchel Papers, General Correspondence Files, Municipal Archives, New York City. Also cited by Rogers, "Screen the Baby, Swat the Fly," 155.

38. *New York Times*, July 23, 1916. The Italians were hardly alone in their resistence to quarantine. See Guenter B. Risse, "Revolt Against Quarantine: Community Responses to the 1916 Polio Epidemic, Oyster Bay, New York," *Transactions and Studies of the College of Physicians of Philadelphia*, 5th Ser., 14 (1992); 23–50.

39. Irving Howe, *World of Our Fathers: The Journey of the East European Jews to America and the Life They Found and Made* (New York: Harcourt Brace Jovanovich, 1976), 149–150. See also Kraut, *Silent Travelers*, 155–165.

40. Edward Alsworth Ross, *The Old World in the New: The Significance of Past and Present Immigration to the American People* (New York: The Century Company, 1914), 289–290. The Jewish physique has long been fascinating to anti-Semites in both Europe and the United States. Sander L. Gilman's research has been path-breaking in its analysis of this obsession. See Sander L. Gilman, "The Jewish Body: A 'Footnote,'" *Bulletin of the History of Medicine* 64 (Winter 1990): 588–602.

41. Valuable historical studies of tuberculosis are: René and Jean Dubos, *The White Plague: Tuberculosis, Man, and Society* (1952; reprint, New Brunswick, N.J.: Rutgers University Press, 1987); J. Arthur Myers, *Captain of All These Men of Death: Tuberculosis Historical Highlights* (St. Louis: Warren H. Green, 1977); Guy P. Youmans, *Tuberculosis* (Philadelphia: Saunders, 1979). A useful study of the public health campaign against TB is Michael E. Teller, *The Tuberculosis Movement: A Public Health Campaign in the Progressive Era* (New York: Greenwood Press, Connecticut, 1988). An intriguing dissertation on the transformation of the tubercular patient's image from the romantic image of the eighteenth and early nineteenth centuries to the impoverished, wasted image of the late-nineteenth- and twentieth-century victim is Nan Marie McMurry, "'And I? I Am in a Consumption': The Tuberculosis Patient, 1780–1930" (Ph.D. diss., Duke University, 1985).

42. The eminent demographer of disease, Thomas McKeown, in his influential volume, *The Modern Rise of Population* (London: Edward Arnold, 1976), concluded that nonmedical factors, particularly improvements in nutrition and other general aspects of the standard of living, contributed to the decline of infectious diseases, including tuberculosis. More recently, however, historian of medicine Leonard G. Wilson has argued that McKeown was mistaken and that declines in TB mortality were a direct result of removing pulmonary tuberculosis, or phthisis, patients from their families and coworkers to the confines of institutions (increasingly, in the United States, to TB sanitariums). See Leonard G. Wilson, "The Historical Decline of Tuberculosis in Europe and America: Its Causes and Significance," *Journal of the History of Medicine and Allied Sciences* 45 (July 1990):366–396; and Wilson, "The Rise and Fall of Tuberculosis in Minnesota: The Role of Infection," *Bulletin of the History of Medicine* 66 (Spring 1992):16–52. Most recently, Barbara Bates has challenged contentions that separating TB patients from those not yet infected sufficiently accounts for declining rates of the

disease, especially in northeastern states with their highly congested urban areas. See Bates, *Bargaining for Life*, 313–327. For more on the issue, see the heated correspondence between Lind Bryder and Leonard Wilson in the *Journal of the History of Medicine and Allied Sciences* 46 (1991):358–368.

43. The data were compiled from European sources by Maurice Fishberg, "The Comparative Pathology of the Jews," *New York Medical Journal* 73 (1901): 540–541; also, Fishberg, "Tuberculosis Among the Jews," *Transactions of the Sixth International Congress on Tuberculosis* (New York: 1908), 3:415–428, also reprinted in *Medical Record*, December 26, 1908.

44. Maurice Fishberg, "The Relative Infrequency of Tuberculosis Among Jews," *American Medicine* 2 (1901): 695–698. Two articles that mention Fishberg's research and the health of Jewish immigrants generally are Deborah Dwork, "Health Conditions of Immigrant Jews on the Lower East Side of New York: 1880–1914," *Medical History* 25 (1981): 1–40, and Jacob Jay Lindenthal, "Abi Gezunt: Health and the Eastern European Jewish Immigrant," *American Jewish History* 70 (June 1981): 420–441.

45. Fishberg may well have been concerned about the genetic component of European racial discourse finding an increasingly large space in American anti-Semitic rhetoric. See Robert Singerman, "The Jew as Racial Alien: The Genetic Component of American Anti-Semitism," in David A. Gerber, ed., *Anti-Semitism in American History* (Urbana: University of Illinois Press, 1986), 103–128. For a discussion of this phenomenon in Europe, see Sander Gilman's *The Jew's Body* (New York: Routledge, 1991).

46. Fishberg's preference for the environmental argument is evident in his articles, such as those on "Girth of the Chest," "Stature," "Nervous Diseases," and "Morbidity" in the *Jewish Encyclopedia*, which was published by Funk and Wagnall's from 1901 to 1906. See Shuly Rubin Schwartz, *The Emergence of Jewish Scholarship in America: The Publication of the "Jewish Encyclopedia"* (Cincinnati: Hebrew Union College Press, 1991), 110–112.

47. Fishberg, "The Relative Infrequency of Tuberculosis Among Jews," 698.

48. Fishberg, "Tuberculosis Among the Jews," 14.

49. Edward Livingston Trudeau, *An Autobiography* (Garden City, N.Y.: Doubleday Page, 1916). For a recent and popular treatment of Trudeau and the Saranac Lake sanitarium, see Mark Caldwell, *The Last Crusade: The War on Consumption, 1862–1954* (New York: Atheneum, 1988).

50. New York City Department of Health, Bureau of Tuberculosis Control, *Tuberculosis in New York City, 1991 Information Summary*, 3, table 2.

51. In October 1992, the *New York Times* ran a five-part series by Michael Specter on the public health threat of new drug-resistant strains of TB and the absence of adequate care facilities because health care professionals had considered the disease conquered. *New York Times*, October 11–15, 1992.

52. Isaac Metzker tells the anecdote in his commentary on a letter to the editor of the *Jewish Daily Forward*'s "Bintel Brief" (Bundle of Letters) column in Metzker, ed., *A Bintel Brief* (Garden City, N.Y.: Doubleday, 1971), 83. Also quoted by Stefan Kanfer, *A Summer World: The Attempt to Build a Jewish Eden in the Catskills, From the Days of the Ghetto to the Rise and Decline of the Borscht Belt* (New York: Farrar, Straus and Giroux, 1989), 52.

53. Dorothy Levenson, *Montefiore: The Hospital as Social Instrument, 1884–1984* (New York: Farrar, Straus and Giroux, 1984), 3.

54. Ibid., 63–86.

55. Ibid., 65.

56. Patient publications from tuberculosis sanitariums offer a unique perspective on immigrants' feelings about their lives, the disease ravishing their bodies, and the institutions caring for them. *Montefiore Echo* 2 (August 1916): 1.

57. Levenson, *Montefiore*, 84.

58. In 1887, the Denver Chamber of Commerce reported that "Colorado is the Mecca of Consumptives, and rightfully; for dry air, equable temperature and continuous sunshine are as yet the most reliable factors in the cure of this [tuberculosis] disease." *Fourth Annual Report of the Denver Chamber of Commerce* (Denver, 1887). The arrival of impoverished Jewish consumptives from eastern cities soon caused apprehension in the non-Jewish community and among the established German-Jewish elite. See Lyle Dorsett and Michael McCarthy, *The Queen City: A History of Denver*, 2nd ed. (Boulder, Colo.: Pruitt Publishing Company, 1986), 176–180, and Robert H. Shikes, *Rocky Mountain Medicine: Doctors, Drugs, and Disease in Early Colorado* (Boulder, Colo.: Johnson Books, 1986), 156–170. A biography of Israeli Prime Minister Golda Meir mentions the political conflict in Denver occasioned by impoverished tubercular Jews. See Ralph G. Martin, *Golda, Golda Meir: The Romantic Years* (New York: Charles Scribner's Sons, 1988), 31. An anecdotal but useful study of Denver's Jewish community and its efforts to cope with its unusual burdens is Ida Libert Uchill, *Pioneers, Peddlers and "Tsadikim"* (Boulder, Colo.: Quality Line Printing, 1957).

59. *First Annual Report of National Jewish Hospital at Denver Colorado* (1900). See Mary Ann Fitzharris, *A Place to Heal: The History of National Jewish Center for Immunology and Respiratory Medicine* (Boulder, Colo.: Johnson Publishing Company, 1989), 1.

60. Ibid.

61. Jeanne Lichtman Abrams is the single most knowledgeable scholar on the history of the JCRS. See Jeanne Lichtman Abrams, "Chasing the Cure: A History of the Jewish Consumptives' Relief Society" (Ph.D. diss., University of Colorado, 1983). She has also written on Anna Hilkowitz, one of the female volunteers for the JCRS; see Abrams, "Unsere Leit (Our People): Anna Hilkowitz and the Development of the East European Jewish Woman Professional in America," *American Jewish Archives* 37 (November 1985): 275–289. Jewish consumptives in Denver often also suffered family dislocation. See Abrams, "'For a Child's Sake': The Denver Sheltering Home for Jewish Children in the Progressive Era," *American Jewish History* 79 (Winter 1989–90): 181–202.

62. Charles Spivak, "The Genesis and Growth of the Jewish Consumptives' Relief Society, I," *The Sanatorium* (January 1907): 6–7.

63. Charles Spivak, "The Genesis and Growth of the Jewish Consumptives' Relief Society, II," *The Sanatorium* (March 1907): 26.

64. Letter to Charles Spivak from Workman's Circle of New York, February 28, 1908, Workman's Circle Folder, Jewish Consumptives' Relief Society Archives, Beck Archives of Rocky Mountain Jewish History, University of Denver.

65. Letter to Charles Spivak from Rochester Workman's Circle, June 6, 1908.

66. Howe, *World of Our Fathers*, 149.

67. Spivak's life has been pieced together by Abrams, "Chasing the Cure," 11–15.

68. *Yiddishe Gazetten*, April 1894, as quoted by Moses Rischin, *The Promised City: New York's Jews, 1870–1914* (1962; reprint, New York: Harper and Row, 1970), 104.

69. *Jewish Outlook* 1 (April 15, 1904): 7, 8.

70. Dr. Philip Hilkowitz, "President's Report," *The Sanatorium Sixth Annual Report* (1910), 38.

71. Rabbi William S. Friedman, "Modern Methods of Fighting Tuberculosis: What the National Jewish Hospital for Consumptives is Doing" (Address delivered before the National Jewish Chautauqua at Atlantic City, New Jersey, July 28, 1905), National Jewish Hospital Archive, Denver, Colorado.

72. Fitzharris, *A Place to Heal*, 15.

73. "Eleventh and Twelfth Annual Reports of the Jewish Consumptives' Relief Society," *The Sanatorium*, 4 (July–December 1916): 68. Also, Abrams, "Chasing the Cure," 95–97. The resolution of the Colorado State Board of Health's fears with a "warning label" is described in Medical Advisory Board Minutes, November 8, 1926, 33, in the Beck Archives.

74. *Jewish Outlook* (October 7, 1904): 6.

75. Dr. Adolph Zederbaum, "Kosher Meat in Jewish Hospitals and Sanatoria," *The Sanatorium* 2 (November 1908): 275, Beck Archives. In 1925, National Jewish finally did establish a kosher kitchen. The cultural tensions embodied in the debate over kashrut took much longer to abate, however.

76. Susan Sontag, *Illness As Metaphor* (New York: Random House, 1977), and Sontag, *AIDS and Its Metaphors* (New York: Farrar, Straus and Giroux, 1988).

77. The author was a guest at the ceremony and witnessed the protest.

78. An excellent example is the video, *Sei Met Ko*, in Haitian French with English subtitles.

79. Many scholars share the notion that disease is socially constructed, but it has been framed with particular clarity in some of Charles Rosenberg's essays, including "Deconstructing Disease," *Reviews in American History* 14 (1986): 110–115; "Disease and Social Order in America," *Millbank Quarterly* 64 (1986): 34–55; "Afterword 1987," 11, in *The Cholera Years*. Also, P. Wright and A. Treacher, eds., *The Problem of Medical Knowledge: Examining the Social Construction of Medicine* (Edinburgh: Edinburgh University Press, 1982).

II

When Epidemic Strikes

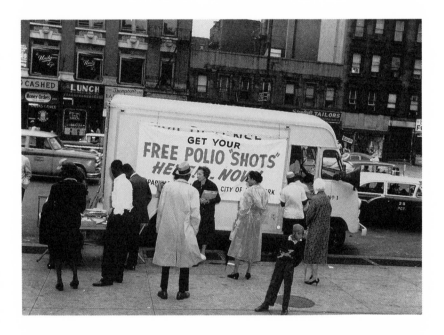

One of two mobile Salk polio vaccination clinics operated by the New York City Department of Health. New York, August 4, 1959. Collection of March of Dimes Birth Defects Foundation.

In a democratic culture, the views of public health officials sometimes come into conflict with deeply held political and cultural beliefs regarding personal rights and civil liberties. Historically, there has been continuous contention over defining the propriety and even the legality of public health interventions necessary to stem disease. For example, should public health have the right to remove people from their homes forcibly and take them to quarantine hospitals? Should officials have the right to mandate the vaccination of schoolchildren over the objections of their parents? What limits should be placed on the police power of health department officials, and when is it appropriate for professionals to override personal liberties? Effective public health practice always entailed both technical and political activities aimed at garnering public trust. Ineffective campaigns to improve health often foundered on the failure of professionals to communicate to a broader public the rationale for programs that intruded on civil rights. Epidemics of smallpox, polio, and AIDS have forced communities to confront the tension between personal liberty and public health.

Historically, smallpox has struck with ferocity, causing death and serious scarring of those who survived. From the early colonial period through the beginning of the twentieth century, sporadic epidemics of the disease struck New York, yet the development of the first truly effective preventive medical techniques—inoculation and later vaccination—along with the successful uses of classic methods of disease containment, through the quarantine of ships and the isolation of infected victims, made smallpox campaigns a model for public health. Today, the disease has been declared vanquished following worldwide campaigns to eradicate it, and international committees are debating whether to dispose of existing laboratory samples of the virus. In the first essay in this section, Judith Leavitt outlines the history of the disease in New York, tracing the city's experience during the last major scare. She illustrates that effective public health campaigns depend on public trust as well as technical and effective medical procedures.

Mobilizing support for public health campaigns includes massive educational efforts. Infantile paralysis, or polio, the focus of the second essay, is perhaps the prime example of an immense twentieth-century public health campaign. It is also an example of some of the limitations of such efforts in the absence of a coherent understanding of the disease's causes and means of prevention. Polio was a fearsome disease that terrified mothers and fathers throughout the first half of the twentieth century and paralyzed a man who became one of the most popular U.S. Presidents, yet the mechanism that caused the disease remained mysterious to the vast majority of the population. The belief that it was a "disease of cleanliness" seemed to contradict basic tenets of both the germ theory and the sanitary models of public health. In the absence of professional agreement and public understanding of the mechanism by which the disease was transmitted, voluntary agencies developed programs that attracted enormous financial support but lacked efficacy in stemming the early epidemics. Even following the development of the vaccines, skepticism remained and was only overcome as the postwar faith in the power of science quelled public and professional suspicion. This story provides one of the most impressive examples of the uses of the laboratory in conquering epidemic diseases.

The final chapter, on the recent history of AIDS, brings us back to some of the questions raised by the history of smallpox. As Bayer tells it, AIDS researchers and scientists have found themselves continually forced to address the public's mistrust of the motivations of politicians and scientists. In less than a decade, professional presentation of the disease has shifted wildly as new information about the modes of transmission and the at-risk populations have been developed. When it was first presented during the early 1980s as a disease of gay men and Haitians, many in the population were taught that they were unthreatened. Later in the decade, public health literature shifted, presenting the disease as a threat to all, irrespective of race, gender, age, and sexual orientation. Among groups most at risk, a history of indifference and sometimes even abuse at the hands of public health professionals led to resistance to the very activities aimed at addressing the AIDS crisis.

Like the smallpox campaigns, the evolving definitions of the disease have to address public fear of the infected as well as the fear of groups identified as high-risk. Unlike smallpox, however, the absence of a recognized treatment, effective vaccine, or commonly agreed upon means of prevention forced public health officials to defend actions that were seen as imminent threats to civil liberties. AIDS, tuberculosis, and other epidemic diseases serve as vicious reminders that public health is and has been part of a deeply political process of negotiation and, when handled poorly, can be forced to weather fierce political storms given the intense political importance of public health within the city. The example of AIDS also reminds us that the sense of security created by earlier biomedical "victories" over infectious disease created problems that are now only too apparent. We now struggle with the heightened expectations created by professionals themselves.

"Be Safe. Be Sure."
New York City's Experience with Epidemic Smallpox

The lines of people stretched as far as the eye could see. Men, women, and children, numbering each day in the thousands, stood for hours, sometimes getting drenched in the rain, as they waited their turn. The mood of the crowds was cheerful for the most part, except when word of delay was passed along the lines; then the police trying to control the masses of people had some difficulty. The people were not in line for tickets to a concert or a World Series game: they queued up to receive free smallpox vaccinations. It was April 1947, and the New Yorkers were responding to a threat of an epidemic of smallpox, a loathsome and often fatal disease that most of them had never seen.

The characteristic rash of the disease had become so rare in New York that doctors misdiagnosed the early cases. Smallpox was so unusual, in fact, that citizens had lost their worry about contracting it, and most New Yorkers in that spring of 1947 had not protected themselves through the sure-preventive vaccination. Only an estimated two million of the city's seven and one half million inhabitants had any degree of immunity. The population was thus at risk to contract the disease if exposed, and possibly to die from it. The danger was real, and health officials recognized it when Dr. Dorothea M. Tolle, the medical superintendent of Willard Parker Hospital, the city's reception point for people with contagious diseases, telephoned the City Health Department on March 28, 1947, and reported two suspected cases of smallpox.

THE 1947 SMALLPOX OUTBREAK

Exposure had arrived, innocently, on March 1 on a cross-country bus that had stopped in Texas, Missouri, Ohio, and Pennsylvania, on its way from Mexico City to New York City. Two passengers on that bus, Mr. and Mrs. Eugene Le Bar, had traveled the whole distance, planning to continue on to Maine. By the time the bus reached New York, however, Eugene Le Bar was not feeling well, and the two delayed their journey and checked in at a midtown Manhattan hotel for a rest. During the hours when Eugene felt well enough, the couple explored the city, walking along Fifth Avenue and stopping in a few

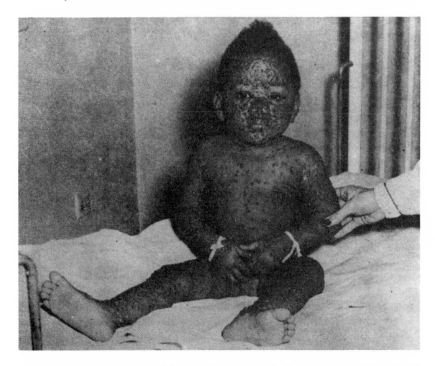

Infant twenty-two months old—smallpox on tenth day after onset. From Israel Weinstein, "An Outbreak of Smallpox in New York City," *American Journal of Public Health* 37 (1947). Copyright © American Public Health Association.

shops. But by March 5, Le Bar felt worse, and he went for help to Bellevue Hospital, where he was admitted to the dermatology service. His condition continued to deteriorate, however, and baffled Bellevue's skin doctors. Le Bar was transferred to Willard Parker Hospital with an unknown but suspected contagious condition. On March 10, Eugene Le Bar died. His doctor's diagnosis was bronchitis with hemorrhages. His wife continued on her way to Maine.

The public knew nothing of these events. Even when Dr. Tolle tentatively diagnosed smallpox in two other patients and reported them to the Health Department on March 28, the news media were not apprised of the situation. At that time, the health officials vaccinated the staff and patients at Willard Parker, isolated the suspected cases, and forwarded specimens from them to the Army Medical School Laboratory in Washington, D.C., for a confirming diagnosis. While they awaited the results of laboratory tests, officials meanwhile tried to establish a link between the two sick people, one a twenty-two-month-old black child from the Bronx and the other a twenty-five-year-old Puerto Rican man from Harlem. They soon established that both had been

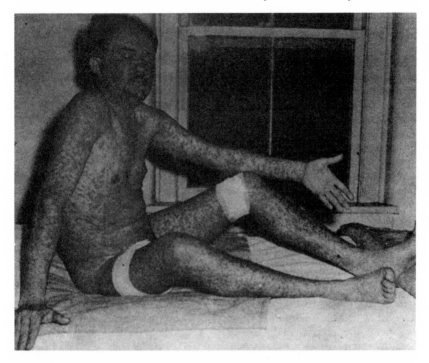

A.—twenty-seven years old—smallpox on the eighth day of the disease. From Israel Weinstein, "An Outbreak of Smallpox in New York City," *American Journal of Public Health* 37 (1947). Copyright © American Public Health Association.

patients at Willard Parker previously, the baby with tonsillitis and the man with mumps, overlapping in time with Eugene Le Bar's admission. Both were unvaccinated. On April 4, the Health Department received back from Washington the laboratory report that matter taken from these patients, and from Le Bar, unmistakably revealed smallpox. On April 5, New Yorkers opened their morning newspapers to learn of their risk.[1]

Health Commissioner Israel Weinstein weighed his words to the press carefully. On the one hand, Dr. Weinstein assured the public that the chances of a full-scale virulent epidemic were "slight." He did not want to promote panic. On the other hand, Weinstein and Hospital Commissioner Edward M. Bernecker called for all who "have never been vaccinated or who have not been vaccinated since childhood to go at once to their doctors to receive this protection."[2] The health officials wanted to give a strong message so that people would actually take the time to gain protection, but not so strong that social order would break down. The motto, repeated over and over again, was "Be safe. Be sure. Get vaccinated." More than four weeks had passed since Le Bar had frequented the downtown hotel, walked the city streets, and lay sick and dying (but not isolated) in two city hospitals. His contacts had had ample time to spread the virus unwittingly but liberally throughout and beyond the five boroughs.

In the days following the initial revelation, the newspapers reported other cases of smallpox, suspected and confirmed. On April 7 a man suffering from smallpox was admitted to Willard Parker Hospital. The next day two more people suspected of having smallpox were hospitalized. On April 13, Mrs. Carmen Acosta, the pregnant wife of one of the earliest sufferers, died at Willard Parker. On April 14 New Yorkers learned that the disease had spread to Dutchess County, by way of a young boy who had brought smallpox to the village of Millbrook from his stay at Willard Parker as a scarlet fever patient. And a case of smallpox traced to New York appeared in Bremerhaven, Germany. Within two weeks of becoming established in New York City, smallpox had infected twelve persons; with each new identification, the health commissioner stepped up his activities. (See Diagram)

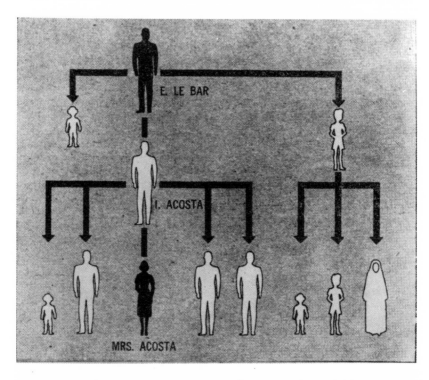

Disease spread from Eugene Le Bar to Ismael Acosta and two children. Acosta in turn infected his wife, who died, and two others. One child who was infected by Le Bar passed virus to two children and a nun in Millbrook, N.Y. Credited to *Life*, in Israel Weinstein, "An Outbreak of Smallpox in New York City," *American Journal of Public Health* 37 (1947).

Efforts to prevent an epidemic from sweeping the city moved in two directions simultaneously. First was the mass vaccination campaign; second was the case-tracing epidemiological work. Health officials saw both as essential to ultimate success.

To encourage everyone to seek a vaccination, the Health Department provided free vaccinations at each of its twenty-one neighborhood health centers and sixty child health stations. The thirteen municipal hospitals provided the service in their out-patient clinics. Once the campaign was in full swing, Weinstein organized free vaccinations at the eighty-four police precincts throughout the city. All public and parochial schools offered vaccinations to their pupils. Many people received their vaccinations from private physicians or at clinics established through labor unions or industry. Mayor William O'Dwyer, amid great publicity, submitted to the procedure while urging his fellow citizens to follow his example. President Harry S. Truman, planning a visit to New York, underwent vaccination as well. The press and radio provided vaccination center schedules and helpful hints for easing the pain of sore arms. Each day the newspapers trumpeted the numbers vaccinated: at the height of the program half a million New Yorkers got their arms scratched with the virus in a single day. In the two weeks following the discovery of smallpox in the city, 5,000,000 New Yorkers had been vaccinated; by the end of one month, with the danger over and the campaign completed, 6,350,000 people had had their arms pricked in the name of disease prevention.[3] More people had been vaccinated in a shorter period of time than ever before in history.

The vaccination campaign owed its success not just to a well-planned and well-executed Health Department response, but also to the federal and local government. Midway through the month of April, the city and private laboratories that had been producing vaccine reached their limit. People waiting in line to be vaccinated were told to come back another time. An emergency call to the navy, army, and the U.S. Public Health Service provided new supplies of the vital fluid. Simultaneously, Mayor O'Dwyer put pressure on the drug companies to produce more and to sell the larger quantities to the city at a cheaper price. Dr. Tom Rivers, a Board of Health member and head of the Rockefeller Institute for Medical Research, advised the mayor during the epidemic. He attended a meeting during which O'Dwyer virtually locked the pharmaceutical representatives into City Hall until they agreed to comply with his demands.[4]

Once the vaccine itself became available in sufficient quantity, another deficit in people power emerged. It took a lot of people, more than the city government had on ready call, to organize and execute a massive vaccination campaign. The Health Department sought volunteer help. At least three thousand individuals came forward to offer aid: many came from the American Red Cross, the Civilian Defense Volunteer Organization, and the American

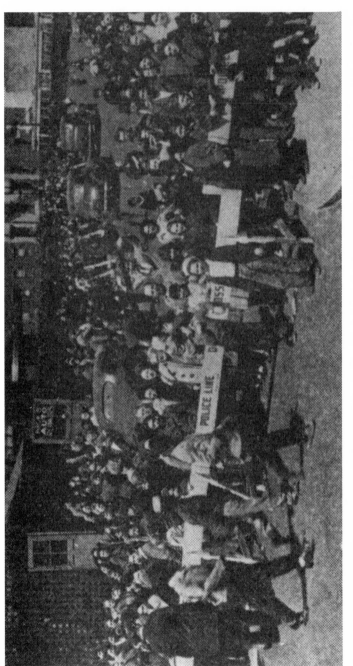

Waiting to be vaccinated, New Yorkers form a line outside of the Brooklyn Headquarters Building of the Department of Health. Credited to *New York News* in Israel Weinstein, "An Outbreak of Smallpox in New York City," *American Journal of Public Health* 37 (1947).

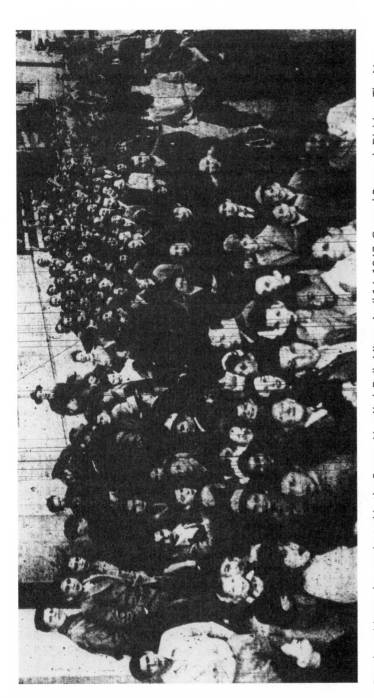

People waiting to be vaccinated in the Bronx. *New York Daily Mirror*, April 14, 1947. General Research Division, The New York Public Library, Astor, Lenox and Tilden Foundations

Women's Voluntary Services. Organizations active during the recent war mobilization quickly reassembled their volunteers to help the nurses and physicians who were galvanized to help puncture citizens' arms.

Widespread public compliance with these efforts can be attributed, in large part, to the postwar period in which the epidemic occurred. Not only were wartime volunteers still available, but the public also retained something of an emergency mentality and easily followed government advice. Furthermore, the city health officials consciously and carefully kept the vaccination program voluntary, appealing to citizens' judgment instead of trying to force compliance, a stance that heightened reasoned responses and kept public panic at a minimum.

In addition to the mass vaccination campaign in 1947, the New York City Health Department initiated a second stage of its smallpox prevention efforts: tracing possible contacts of the people who had confirmed cases of the disease. Because Eugene Le Bar had traveled throughout the country during the period when he was infectious, and because bus passengers, hotel patrons, hospital patients, and others with whom he might have had contact were spread throughout the country as well as beyond its borders by the time the danger became known, a coordinated effort among government agencies at the local, state, and federal level became necessary. In order to make sure that smallpox did not spread far from this target case, all people who were exposed to Le Bar or the other people already identified and hospitalized had to be vaccinated and observed for a full twenty-one days. Hundreds of people had stayed in the (unnamed) midtown hotel during the five days the Le Bars were there. They were scattered around the country and had to be traced and watched. Mrs. Le Bar herself was followed to Maine by the U.S. Public Health Service. All the people who had gotten on and off the bus in Texas, Missouri, Ohio, and Pennsylvania needed to be found and warned. Anyone who had been a patient or visited a patient at Bellevue or Willard Parker during the critical dates had to be located and protected. What about the people the Le Bars and their contacts had passed on the street or jostled in the subway? The task was enormous. That it proceeded systematically and methodically is a testament to how far public health in general and smallpox control in particular had progressed in New York by the middle of the twentieth century.

HISTORY OF SMALLPOX IN NEW YORK CITY

Smallpox had a long history on Manhattan island. It first appeared during the Dutch occupation, probably in 1649, and recurred throughout the colonial period.[5] In the first half of the nineteenth century, smallpox seemed endemic, although it was not one of the city's major killers. During the second half of the nineteenth century, smallpox appeared more sporadically, but when it flared up its impact could be severe. In the 1870s it sometimes accounted for more than 1,000 deaths yearly; it resumed its devastation for a few years during the 1880s and again briefly in the 1890s. At the very beginning of the twentieth century—in 1901 and 1902—New York suffered another epidemic, during which over 2,500 people contracted the disease and more than 700 of them died. But then it seemed to be finished. Two cases were discovered in 1922, six in 1925, and one more in 1939: they seemed anomalous to a population already feeling beyond reach of smallpox's dangers. It was the mirage of safety, possibly, that led many New Yorkers not to get vaccinated before a threat reappeared in April 1947, and the weight of previous experience that allowed them to accept the medical protection readily when offered it.

From the colonial period through the creation of the Metropolitan Board of Health in 1866 and into the twentieth century, New York confronted issues in disease control that had severely tested both medical and civic authority. In the process the city developed modes of disease control that were acceptable to most New Yorkers and effective in coping with epidemic emergencies. It is worth examining two of the issues that arose historically relative to smallpox in order to comprehend the meaning of the triumphant show of private and public cooperation in 1947. The first concerns the safety and efficacy of variolation and later vaccination as preventives to this disease; the second concerns governmental authority.

Smallpox always elicited a public response when it appeared: it was a horrible disease that could not be ignored. Succumbing to the infection, a sufferer felt flulike symptoms of headache, fever, chills, and nausea; later, in the fair-skinned, a scarlet color crept over the body. Then the victim developed red spots, usually more densely on the face and extremities, which evolved from flat to raised pimples, finally blistering into oozing pustules. In addition to the terrifying outward manifestation, the disease ravaged inside the body, attacking the throat, lungs, heart, liver, and intestines, sometimes causing convulsions, hemorrhages, or delirium. On the average, about one-quarter of the people attacked by smallpox died; lucky victims survived the horror and watched the pustules crust over and the scabs drop off, leaving scars, lifelong reminders of their ordeal. People with smallpox shed literally millions of the disease's viruses into the air; they remained infectious from just before the rash appeared until the scabs disappeared, a period of about three weeks.[6] It is no wonder that when smallpox appeared in a community, inhabitants rushed to try to protect themselves.

Limiting the Disease

Before the eighteenth century, New Yorkers could do little more than quarantine in the harbor ships containing smallpox sufferers and isolate those people who caught the disease on land. In 1721, however, another alternative, inoculation, was tried in Boston, and its use spread southward in time for the epidemic that struck New York City in 1731.[7] Long used in Africa and Asia, inoculation with matter from a smallpox pustule, when introduced under the skin of a person who had never had the disease, seemed to protect effectively against a virulent attack. The procedure, known technically as variolation, produced a mild case of smallpox but only rarely led to death. It produced, as did smallpox acquired naturally, lifetime immunity. In 1732, the procedure appeared to be quite popular in the New York area: 160 people submitted to inoculation in Jamaica in that year, and only 1 of them died, a significantly smaller number than the expected one-quarter of naturally acquired cases.[8]

Variolation had its drawbacks, unfortunately. Not only was there a small chance of death in people who might never have contracted the natural disease, but inoculation with a case of smallpox, no matter how mild, produced a person just as infectious as someone who had contracted the disease through the ordinary routes. Thus, communities that adopted inoculation policies risked spreading cases of smallpox much more widely than might have occurred had they not started the practice. In so doing, officials put people who did not choose to protect themselves through variolation (from religious beliefs, for example, that prohibited tampering with God's will) at greater risk of catching the infection.

Although hotly contested in its early years, variolation rapidly gained advocates, and its use spread throughout the English colonies. Benjamin Franklin, having lost a child to naturally acquired smallpox in 1736, became one of its most ardent supporters. In his autobiography he wrote his feelings about his son's death: "A fine boy of four years old, by the smallpox, taken in the common way. I long regretted him, and still regret that I had not given it to him by inoculation. This I mention for the sake of parents who omit that operation, on the supposition that they should never forgive themselves, if a child died under it, my example showing that the regret may be the same either way, and therefore the safer should be chosen."[9] Other parents used arguments similar to Franklin's to convince themselves to inoculate their children, and soon more people caught smallpox from the knife than from exposure. The more people were inoculated with the disease, the more rapidly it spread; the more it spread, the more people would try to protect themselves through inoculation. The infection was thus kept alive by inoculation; it also was prevented from wreaking its worst ravages.

The cycle of infection and variolation was broken in 1801, when Drs. Valentine Seaman and David Hosack made available in New York a new procedure, imported from Great Britain.[10] Vaccination—inoculation with cowpox matter—was far safer than introducing smallpox directly; it effectively provided immunity from smallpox but did not lead to its dissemination. Vaccination quickly replaced variolation as the procedure of choice for those seeking protection from smallpox.

One of the ironies of American medical history is that despite the availability of effective and safe vaccination, smallpox continued for almost 150 years periodically to scourge communities around the country. This is in great part because of enemies of vaccination who worked hard to convince people that the procedure was dangerous and ineffective: dangerous because vicious infections or other diseases such as syphilis could be transferred from one person to another through the procedure and ineffective because cases of smallpox could be traced to people who thought themselves protected by vaccination.[11] New York harbored its share of the so-called antivaccinationists, who were busy in the nineteenth century trying to convince people not to submit to the procedure. They were often successful in turning people against vaccination. During the New York City epidemic of 1853 and 1854, for example, one mother deliberately exposed her four children to smallpox instead of vaccinating them, "in order that they might have the disease at once, and thus relieve her from the anxiety." Three of the children died.[12]

The antivaccinationists spoke directly to a concern that all citizens, and especially immigrant groups, harbored about violations of personal liberty. Many people had come to America to escape governmental tyranny: was governmental repression reemerging on these shores in the guise of "free" vaccinations? Seeing the issue in these terms, and fearing vaccination as a first step toward greater governmental intervention in private lives and decision-making, many people joined the ranks of the antivaccinationists and resisted public programs aimed to protect them from smallpox.

New York's antivaccinationists stepped up their activity after the Metropolitan Board of Health was formed in 1866.[13] An Anti-Vaccination League was begun in 1885, and it challenged the Board of Health to debate the "evils of vaccination."[14] The board refused, but groups around the city did use their meetings to discuss the issues raised in the vaccination controversy. The Society of Medical Jurisprudence and State Medicine, for example, discussed smallpox at one of its meetings, agreeing among themselves that vaccination was "an excellent thing."[15] During the virulent epidemic of 1893–94, when health officials brandished their power to detain forcibly any who refused vaccination, the Anti-Compulsory Vaccination League, a Brooklyn-based group, successfully sued the Brooklyn Department of Health. On appeal the suit was overthrown, but the incident put before the public the issue of infringement of personal liberty, which the antivaccinationists emphasized. Thereafter New York health officials were wont to highlight educational persuasion instead of their police powers.[16]

One of the reasons the antivaccinationists were successful in their campaign to convince some people not to undergo vaccination was the truth of their arguments about the risks of the procedure as it was practiced in the nineteenth century. Indeed, many doctors, so-called regulars and irregulars alike, agreed that vaccination as it was practiced could transmit other diseases and lead to a false sense of security. Some practitioners still used "humanized" virus during the second half of the nineteenth century, matter taken from the pustules of inoculated humans, which could carry with it the added danger of infecting recipients with other diseases, such as syphilis. If transmitted through too many people, the virus lost its powers of inducing immunity. Most inoculators by the last third of the century used bovine matter, which they considered safer as well as more effective than the humanized material, but which, when kept too long, also gave minimal protection against smallpox. Furthermore, the inoculation procedure itself could be a cause for worry. Scarification, puncture, or abrasion prepared the skin for the introduction of the viral matter from the "point" on which it was stored. If inoculators were in a hurry, or if they were not sufficiently trained, they might fail to clean the puncture site adequately or use a single point to lance many people. It was not surprising that many laypeople found it difficult to interpret their degree of safety in the face of varied practices and conflicting information.[17]

The Politics of Prevention

The questions raised by the uncertainty of smallpox inoculation practices in the second half of the nineteenth century significantly involved the issue of state power. Should the government step in to regulate the practice of vaccination itself, thus insuring its safety and quelling citizen doubts? Should it at the same time insist that citizens must protect themselves, thus making vaccination compulsory? What level of government had legal authority to regulate these practices, and how far could it impinge on personal liberty? Turning now to this issue of the authority of the government, we can examine the evolution of public authority to protect the public's health, specifically through smallpox prevention. Through this example, we can begin to understand how citizens, working through their worries about possible violation of individual liberties, were convinced to allow the government to take control to the extent witnessed during the 1947 smallpox epidemic in New York City.

The year before the formation of the New York Metropolitan Board of Health in 1866, Dr. J. M. Toner, a noted physician and writer, published a paper on the "propriety and necessity of compulsory vaccination," in which he challenged physicians and health officials to use their powers to protect the public health through vaccination.[18] He maintained that it was the duty of government to protect the health of its citizens if they would not do it themselves, and that officials should "secure effective vaccine protection to every person, without distinction, residing within the sphere of their authority." Parents, too, had duties in Toner's plan. He insisted that vaccination was as important for parents to provide for children as were food and clothing: "failure to provide protection against the smallpox seems to be more maliciously wicked than to neglect either food or clothing, as the former may not only cause the death of the child, but be the means of spreading disease and death among many others." Thus, holding parents responsible but putting on government the burden of providing the services and enforcing vaccination, Toner's proposal set the stage for debate for the rest of the century.[19]

The issues Toner raised were discussed widely in the medical and lay literature of the second half of the nineteenth century. It became essential for health departments to devise strategies to try to prevent smallpox and to define the role of the state unambiguously. In New York, before the 1866 Metropolitan Health Act was passed, health officers repeatedly voiced their frustration about their lack of authority to handle smallpox emergencies. In 1862, for example, officials sent 320 people to the Smallpox Hospital on Blackwell Island, but another 83 refused to go and could not be pressured. In 1865, the press noted that "there is no adequate legal power to prevent [smallpox] spreading. . . . [P]ersons taken with this disease are allowed to travel in the cars and stages which are constantly running in the principal thoroughfares."[20] The *New York Times* concluded, "The prophylactic against smallpox is vaccination; but this end cannot be attained except through the agency of strong laws energetically enforced."[21] The seemingly intractable problem was one of the factors moving New Yorkers to support the imposition of stronger health authority.

The first response of the more powerful Board of Health was to regularize the production and accessibility of smallpox vaccine. In its first *Annual Report*, the new board noted that the recent dispensing of 70,000 vaccinations free of charge had resulted in a mild epidemic (35 people had died of smallpox in the board's first eight months of operation) and that city physicians hoped that their success would "lead to the adoption of systematic methods for the vaccination of all children and unprotected persons."[22] Indeed, the health ordinances adopted in the early months of the board's operation provided "that every person, being the parent or guardian, or having the care, custody or control of any minor or other individual, shall . . . cause and procure such minor or individual to be so promptly, frequently and effectively vaccinated, that such minor or individual shall not take, or be liable to take, the smallpox."[23]

Despite these firm words and intentions, New York officials did not portray their vaccination policy then or later in the century as compulsory. Insisting that "compulsory" measures could be enforced only under "imperial" governments, and that New York City's policy was not compulsory because such rules "would result in antagonism to the work, which would defeat the object," health officials seemed to be obfuscating reality. Not only did the board actively encourage vaccination and provide it free to all who wanted it, it also cooperated with the Board of Education in enforcing an ordinance that made vaccination a prerequisite to school attendance at all schools in the city. By the time of the 1947 smallpox scare, New York was one of only twelve states to require such school-related vaccination even in the absence of a threat of smallpox. During the years when smallpox actually threatened the city, the board went much further, insisting that all inhabitants be vaccinated or else submit to isolation measures to protect those around them.[24]

From 1866 to the beginning of the new century, New York tested and refined its smallpox strategies. In addition to establishing school-based programs and offering free vaccination to all, the board instituted house-to-house vaccination visits in 1871. The same year, the board systematically began to remove to the Smallpox Hospital all those suffering from smallpox who could not be "properly isolated" at home.[25] Yet smallpox recurred. In the words of one observer, its continued presence was due to "the positive refusal of large numbers of our foreign population to submit to vaccination."[26] Limits in budget and personnel left the health department incapable of full-scale actions.

The legal status of vaccination rested on prevailing, and by the twentieth century increasingly unanimous, medical opinion. In the words of sanitarian M. J. Rosenau, "Vaccination affords a high degree of immunity to the individual, and well-nigh perfect protection to the community. To remain unvaccinated is selfish in that by so doing a person steals a certain measure of protection from the community on account of the barrier of vaccinated persons around him."[27] Rosenau advocated compulsory vaccination. Yet he and probably most other Americans by the early twentieth century did not equate "compulsory" with forcible policies. The question of the invasion of personal liberties of citizens—the degree to which such liberties could be abridged by government in the name of protecting the public health—remained of paramount concern. A policy mandating vaccination was not the same as one forcing citizens to undergo such a procedure.

Vaccination requirements as promulgated by state legislatures, municipal ordinances, and school board regulations emanated from the police power of the states. They were not delegated to the federal government in the Constitution. State legislatures could require vaccination of all citizens under conditions that they stipulated, or they could delegate such power to municipalities or other governmental bodies such as boards of health. Throughout the second half of the nineteenth century, the extent of police powers was becoming understood largely through court rulings. Public health officials and private citizens continued to debate the constitutionality of compulsory vaccination, a debate especially spurred on by antivaccination groups. The issues were ultimately settled in law if not in everyone's mind by a United States Supreme Court decision, *Jacobson* v. *Massachusetts*, handed down in 1905.[28]

The differences between compulsory and forcible measures in vaccination regulations became clear in Justice Harlan's opinion. The case involved a citizen of the Commonwealth of Massachusetts, Henning Jacobson, who did not want to submit to vaccination. The state legislature had empowered boards of health to require vaccination if an epidemic threatened. When smallpox appeared in the city, the Cambridge Board of Health adopted such a regulation and ordered all inhabitants to be vaccinated. Jacobson argued that the ruling was inconsistent with the spirit of the Constitution and violated his individual rights. Justice Harlan and six of his colleagues on the Supreme Court thought otherwise: "The liberty secured by the Constitution of the United States to every person within its jurisdiction does not import an absolute right in each person to be, at all times and in all circumstances, wholly freed from restraint. There are manifold restraints to which every person is necessarily subject for the common good. . . . Real liberty for all could not exist under the operation of the principle which recognizes the right of each individual person to use his own, whether in respect of his person or his property, regardless of the injury that may be done to others." Harlan based his judgment, in part, on a prior New York case in which the exclusion of children from school unless vaccinated had been upheld in those instances in which smallpox threatened the community.[29]

The most important issue for Justice Harlan was the danger to other people posed by individuals or groups who would not cooperate with health officials. But there were limits to how far the state could go in protecting the public health. Nowhere in this decision, or in any other, did the court rule that people could be forcibly vaccinated against their will. As legal expert James Tobey concluded from his analysis of vaccination laws, "Compulsory vaccination means that all persons may be required to submit to vaccination for the common good, and if they refuse . . . they may be arrested, fined, imprisoned, quarantined, isolated, or excluded from school . . . but they cannot be forcibly vaccinated, desirable as such a procedure might be from the standpoint of public health protection."[30] Individual liberty and public health could be protected simultaneously under compulsory vaccination provisions, but there were limits on each.

Resolution of the seeming incompatibility between individual liberty and public health at the beginning of the twentieth century made it much easier for subsequent boards of health to develop and effectuate policies to control smallpox. Although New York City was not threatened by smallpox again in a major way after 1901, it did encounter a few threats. In June 1911, for example, a woman arrived in New York from Washington sick with smallpox. Her physician reported the case to the Health Department, which promptly removed the woman to an isolation hospital and then launched its vaccination efforts. Seventeen police officers and fifteen doctors arrived in the West Side neighborhood armed with vaccination tools. The newspaper reported their efforts: "The work began on the ground floor of each building that none of those on the upper floors should escape. All the apartments were then visited in turn and the tenants informed of the danger of infection. . . . Many of the grownups objected to being vaccinated. . . . In families where there were young children, however, there was little opposition on the part of parents."[31]

Three years later a man appeared at the Health Department office suffering from smallpox. The elevator and the rooms he had visited were fumigated and all employees were revaccinated.[32] The existence of a few cases of smallpox in 1925 elicited a citywide vaccination campaign, headed by Mayor Hylan, who was vaccinated in front of the press. The warning Health Commissioner Monaghan issued in that year could have been repeated in 1947: "It is a curious consequence of the efficacy of vaccination that numberless communities have almost forgotten that there is such a thing as smallpox, and many physicians never have seen a case of it. Therein lies the danger at present, for the malady is far from extinct, though it ought to be and might have been if universal vaccination had been practiced for a sufficient period all over the country."[33]

In many respects, the experience in 1925 predicted what would follow twenty-two years later. The city contributed extra funds for a wide-scale vaccination campaign, vaccination remained voluntary, businesses offered the procedure to employees, and publicity was widespread. The *New York Times* editorialized that any inhabitants who had not been vaccinated "ought to feel a sense of duty unperformed." The newspaper revealed the dangers when it told of one undiagnosed smallpox victim who had traveled to his physician in a crowded subway train; the only way to protect against such unwitting transmission of the disease, the paper concluded, was to submit to "the most trivial of 'operations.'"[34] Volunteers from organizations such as the Association for Improving the Condition of the Poor, the New York Diet Kitchen Association, the Maternity Center Association, and the Henry Street Settlement helped. The Health Department put especial effort into vaccinating schoolchildren, giving each pupil a blue-and-white button to wear: on it the seal of the city was surrounded with the words, "I am protected by vaccination. Are you?"[35] When the feared epidemic did not appear, his political foes accused the health commissioner of creating the emergency to produce jobs for his friends. But threatened epidemics and outbreaks elsewhere in the country in 1925 provided evidence of New York's prudent behavior.[36]

A Balance of Power

Both the efficacy of the vaccination procedure and an understanding of the limits of governmental authority were necessary prerequisites to successful epidemic smallpox prevention and control. New Yorkers, and Americans in general, learned through the ups and downs of the nineteenth- and twentieth-century experiences that vaccination, if the practice could be carefully controlled (which became significantly easier after the federal government regulated vaccine production in 1902), was safe. Epidemics could be forestalled. Local government and health departments had important roles to play in such epidemic control; in fact, eradication of the threat of epidemics could not occur without effective governmental actions.

The specific actions planned by Health Commissioner Weinstein and his advisors in 1947 were telling. Despite broad, well-defined police powers that could have been invoked in the instance of a threat from smallpox, these health officials decided to emphasize voluntary vaccination. Furthermore, they relied heavily on public education through the press and the radio to convince the public of its duty, and they effectively utilized contacts with health officials at various levels of government throughout the country to tackle the tough job of case tracing. Tom Rivers's account of how Mayor O'Dwyer, behind the scenes, strong-armed the companies producing the vaccine to get them to agree to produce the necessary quantities and charge reasonable rates indicates that interagency cooperation was not always immediately forthcoming. But it did materialize under strategically placed pressure.

No doubt contributing to the successes of 1947 was the fact that the scare occurred in the aftermath of the Second World War. New Yorkers had already become accustomed to regulations that affected the behavior of the whole population, from food rationing to blackout drills. Throughout the war period, health officials had urged vaccination (although most people did not seem to have complied with this) because of the possibility of mass evacuation and the potential dangers from new environments.[37] Wartime voluntary agencies had been active and could be quickly reassembled.

Perhaps most important in the 1947 effort, health officials encouraged a network of citizen conduct and volunteer activity to support their efforts, thus reaching into the community to sustain the prevention work, gaining cooperation without requiring it. With the power of the law behind him, Weinstein did not need to use it. New Yorkers had learned through a long history with smallpox how devastating the disease could be and how vaccination could provide protection against its worst ravages. People had become accustomed to the exercise of governmental authority. On its part, the Board of Health had learned to value citizen cooperation and to seek it in broadly acceptable ways, largely through publicity and convincing argument.

In assessing the successes of April 1947, Weinstein made note of what might have happened. If the experience had mirrored the 1901–1902 epidemic, with the same case and mortality rate, New York would have reported 4,310 cases of smallpox and 902 deaths. By comparison, the statistics of 12 cases and 2 deaths looked fine. The health commissioner spread the credit widely, thanking the press and radio, his staff, the nurses, other city employees, and the mayor. Most of all, he credited the "intelligent cooperation of the public and the generosity of private physicians and volunteer workers," without whom, he thought, "it would have been impossible to have achieved this remarkable record."[38] He was right.

Notes

I am grateful for the timely research assistance of Sarah A. Leavitt and Nancy Ralph.

1. The events are reconstructed from the *New York Times* and the *Daily Mirror* from April 1947. For a particularly vivid account of the epidemic, see Berton Roueché, "A Man From Mexico," which first appeared in the pages of *The New Yorker*, reprinted in *Eleven Blue Men* (New York: Berkley Medallion Books, 1965), 91–108.

2. Quotation from the *Daily Mirror*, April 6, 1947, 5. The relationship between the Health Department and the press is described in Karl Pretshold and Carolyn C. Sulzer, "Speed, Action and Candor: The Public Relations Story of New York's Smallpox Emergency," *Channels* 25 (September 1947): 3–6.

3. Israel Weinstein submitted his report to the mayor on May 11, giving the statistics: 1.6 million had received their vaccinations at public and private hospitals; 1.9 million at Health Department clinics and police stations; 1.2 million received vaccinations at clinics at their place of work or labor union; one million from private physicians, and 650,000 in the city's schools. See the *New York Times,* May 12, 1947. Typical during the campaign was vaccination of 200,000 people a day. This number represented the usual number of vaccinations in a whole year of Health Department work. See also Israel Weinstein, "An Outbreak of Smallpox in New York City," *American Journal of Public Health* 37 (1947): 1376–1384.

4. *Tom Rivers: Reflections on a Life in Medicine and Science*, An Oral History Memoir prepared by Saul Benison (Cambridge: MIT Press, 1967), 385–388. Rivers did not think highly of Israel Weinstein's ability to administer New York's Health Department.

5. John Duffy, *A History of Public Health in New York City, 1625–1866* (New York: Russell Sage Foundation, 1968). This book and Duffy's second volume, *A History of Public Health in New York City, 1866–1966* (New York: Russell Sage Foundation, 1974), provided the background for this historical discussion of New York's experience with smallpox.

6. An excellent book describing modern smallpox, with a lengthy historical section, is C. W. Dixon, *Smallpox* (London: J. and A. Churchill Ltd., 1962). See also Donald R. Hopkins, *Princes and Peasants: Smallpox in History* (Chicago: University of Chicago Press, 1983).

7. For an excellent account of the controversy over inoculation in Boston, see John B. Blake, "The Inoculation Controversy in Boston, 1721–1722," *New England Quarterly* 25 (1952): 489–506; reprinted in Judith Walzer Leavitt and Ronald L. Numbers, eds., *Sickness and Health in America; Historical Readings*, 2nd ed. rev. (Madison: University of Wisconsin Press, 1985), 347–355.

8. Duffy, *Public Health in New York City, 1625–1866*, 55.

9. Quoted in Francis R. Packard, *History of Medicine in the United States* (New York: Paul B. Hoeber, 1931),1:79.

10. The story of Jenner's discovery and the introduction of vaccination into the United States can be read in Hopkins, *Princes and Peasants*; Genevieve Miller, *The Adoption of Inoculation for Smallpox in England and France* (Philadelphia: University of Pennsylvania Press, 1957); John Blake, *Benjamin Waterhouse and the Introduction of Vaccination* (Philadelphia: University of Pennsylvania Press, 1957); and O. E. Winslow, *A Destroying Angel* (Boston: Houghton Mifflin, 1974).

11. Antivaccinationists can be followed in Martin Kaufman, "The American Anti-vaccinationists and Their Arguments," *Bulletin of the History of Medicine* 41 (1967): 463–478, and in Judith Walzer Leavitt, *The Healthiest City: Milwaukee and the Politics of Health Reform* (Princeton: Princeton University Press, 1982).

12. Quoted from J. C. Hutchinson, "On Vaccination and the Causes of the Prevalence of Small-Pox in New York in 1853–4," *New York Journal of Medicine* 12 (1854): 349–368, in Hopkins, *Princes and Peasants*, 269–270.

13. The story of the creation of the Metropolitan Board of Health is well told in Gert H. Brieger, "Sanitary Reform in New York City: Stephen Smith and the Passage of the Metropolitan Health Bill," *Bulletin of the History of Medicine* 40 (1966): 407–429, reprinted in Leavitt and Numbers, *Sickness and Health in America*, 399–413; and in Duffy, *History of Public Health in New York City, 1625–1866*, 540–571.

14. *New York Times*, October 27, 1885.

15. *New York Times*, November 13, 1885.

16. The incident is described in Duffy, *A History of Public Health in New York City, 1625–1866*, 153–154. At the same time as this legal action, New Yorkers learned of the smallpox troubles in Milwaukee, during which citizens rioted in the streets to object to health department policies about vaccination, and the health commissioner was impeached. See Leavitt, *The Healthiest City: Milwaukee*; and *Leslie's Weekly Illustrated Newspaper* 79 (September 27, 1894): 207. The *New York Times* frequently referred to the antivaccinationists as "public enemies"; See, for example, May 6, 1914.

17. For a contemporary account of the vaccination procedure, see W. A. Hardaway, *Essentials of Vaccination; a Compilation of Facts Relating to Vaccine Inoculation and Its Influence in the Prevention of Smallpox* (Chicago: Jansen, McClury and Company, 1882). See also a lengthy discussion of nineteenth-century practices in Dixon, *Smallpox*, 249–295.

18. J. M. Toner, "A Paper on the Propriety and Necessity of Compulsory Vaccination," *Transactions of the American Medical Association* 16 (1865): 307–330.

19. Quotations from ibid., 314, 317. See also William H. Richardson, "Smallpox in New York City, with Some Statistics and Remarks on Vaccination," *Transactions of the New York State Medical Society* (1865), 143–156.

20. *New York Times*, April 29, 1865.

21. Ibid.

22. [First] *Annual Report of the Metropolitan Board of Health, 1866* (Albany: Van Benthuysen & Sons' Steam Printing House, 1867), 309.

23. Ibid., 706.

24. See, for example, the *New York Times*, January 24, 1863. In 1862 the Board of Education passed a bylaw regulating vaccination for schoolchildren, which was endorsed by the health department. To trace vaccination laws, consult William Fowler, "Principal Provisions of Smallpox Vaccination Laws and Regulations in the United States," *Public Health Reports* 56 (January 1941): 167–189; Clark Bell, "Compulsory Vaccination; Should it Be Enforced in Law?" *Journal of the American Medical Association* 28 (January 9, 1897): 49–53; James A. Tobey, *Public Health Law* (New York: The Commonwealth Fund, 1947), 233–250; and the various Annual Reports of the Board of Health. The quotations are from the *Annual Report* (1866), 310, and Bell, "Compulsory Vaccinations," 49.

25. *New York Times*, March 16, 23, 1871. Throughout the 1871–1873 epidemic, newspapers were filled with stories of the terrible conditions within the Smallpox Hospital. Exposés and accusations filled pages of newsprint; the Board of Health tried to dissociate itself from the institution, which was run by the Commissioner of Charities and Corrections, and the issue emerged as highly political. Control was transferred to the Board of Health in 1874.

26. *New York Times*, May 30, 1875.

27. Milton J. Rosenau, *Preventive Medicine and Hygiene*, 6th ed. (New York: D. Appleton-Century, 1935), 21.

28. 197 U.S. 11. On this issue, consult Hampton L. Carson, "The Legal Aspects of Vaccination," *New York Medical Journal* 89 (1909): 106–111. See also Tobey, *Public Health Law*, 238–240; the decision is reproduced in its entirety on pages 359–375 and the quotations here are from that printing.

29. *Viemeister v. White* (1904), 179 N.Y. 235; cited in Tobey, *Public Health Law*, 239.

30. Tobey, *Public Health Law*, 240.

31. *New York Times*, June 25, 1911.

32. *New York Times*, June 13, 1914.

33. Quoted in the *New York Times*, May 16, 1925.

34. *New York Times*, June 4, 1925.

35. *New York Times*, August 9, 1925.

36. See, for example, John P. Koehler, "How Milwaukee Aborted its Smallpox Epidemic," *Wisconsin Medical Journal* 24 (1925): 324.

37. See, for example, *New York Times*, April 27, 1942, referring to directives issued by the health department.

38. Weinstein, "An Outbreak of Smallpox," 1381. See also the *Report of the Department of Health City of New York for the Years 1941–1948* (New York: Department of Health, 1949).

A Disease of Cleanliness: Polio in New York City, 1900–1990

AN IMMIGRANT DIRT DISEASE, 1900–1920

"We are now in the midst of a spreading epidemic of infantile paralysis," William Harvey Young wrote to his wife during the summer of 1916. "The best Drs. of the city are on the job, and in spite of all they can do the cases increase, and the rate of mortality still remains very high." Young, an assistant pastor of a Methodist church, was teaching Bible school in New York City while his wife and infant son visited her parents' home in Cameron, Missouri. "I keep telling the children," he continued, "[about] the advice that is printed in the papers each day, and will get them to be as clean and as careful as possible. But of course it is fortunate that the little fellow is not where it is to endanger him. . . . Today I saw a dozen babies. . . . How I wish they could have the fresh air like Harvey has it."[1]

Epidemic polio, first known as infantile paralysis, was a frightening disease. Hundreds of cases—almost all of them children under five—began to appear in the 1880s in northern Europe and then in North America. In 1907 the number of known polio cases in New York City reached over 1,000, but because polio was not an officially reportable disease until 1911, many mild cases went unrecognized by parents and physicians. In June 1916 epidemic polio reappeared, fiercer than ever; five months later, 27,000 cases of polio had been reported by twenty-six states, with 6,000 deaths. New York City had the largest single incidence of the disease with over 8,900 cases, 2,400 deaths, and a mortality rate of more than one child in four.[2] New York City remained a center for polio epidemics for the next four decades. In this study of polio in New York I argue that the city's changing experiences of the disease were influenced by a shifting public perception of its victims. Initially seen as a disease of unsanitary living and immigrants, polio had become a middle-class disease by the 1930s, a "danger to all." It was not until the 1960s that the city's use of the Salk and Sabin polio vaccines brought the disease under control.

In 1916 frightened parents sought expert advice from public officials and prominent medical experts. Scientists at the Rockefeller Institute for Medical Research in New York City, a private research institute, studied the polio virus through its appearance in experimental monkeys; clinicians at the institute's hospital studied human victims. Lesions found in the brain and spinal cord in autopsy examinations led researchers to call the disease poliomyelitis, an inflammation of the gray matter of the spinal cord. The term *poliomyelitis* was at first used only by scientists and doctors; the shortened version, *polio*, became common among the general public by the 1940s.

Unfortunately, despite the Rockefeller Institute's work and the public's rising expectations of science and scientists, most physicians in New York were unable to combat polio with much more than general hygienic advice. They warned parents not to allow their children to play with unknown or sick children and to avoid crowds and public gatherings such as movie theaters and amusement parks. Many families fled the city, and neighboring communities responded by posting signs warning that children from New York City were not welcome. Residents of Setauket, Long Island, put up a placard reading "Warning.—We are informed that families from the infected parts of New York City and Brooklyn are offering high prices for rooms and houses here. While we sympathize fully with those who are suffering from this dread disease, infantile paralysis, we certainly should be very careful to whom we extend the hospitality of our village, that the dread disease may not make its appearance here."[3] In one possibly anti-Semitic response, ninety-eight Jewish immigrants from New York City who were feared to be carrying the infection were quarantined for three weeks by a New Jersey community.[4]

Although scientists had been studying polio in the early years of the century, they were still unable to explain many of the distinctive characteristics of the disease. Most agreed that polio was caused by a tiny germ or virus. Its spread was not typical of a contagious disease: sometimes it attacked only one child in a family or in a neighborhood. Furthermore, although children in tenement slums were attacked, clean, well-nourished children from middle-class families were also polio victims. Epidemiologists who studied the disease found a higher proportion of cases in suburban neighborhoods where native-born American families lived than in overcrowded city tenements filled with recent immigrants from southern and eastern Europe. Despite this evidence that the infection crossed class and ethnic boundaries, medical researchers were convinced that polio was a dirt disease carried by immigrant children.

City health officials engaged in active, visible efforts to control the spread of the 1916 epidemic and the ensuing public panic: they placarded infected houses, sent suspected cases to the city's infectious-disease hospitals, and enforced city sanitary regulations for housekeepers and food retailers. The places targeted by city officials were primarily immigrant neighborhoods. Officials monitored immigrant festivals, working-class block parties, and public playgrounds. The New York City Health Department canceled the annual three-day celebration of the Italian feast day of Our Lady of Mount Carmel.[5]

Health leaflets, translated into Italian, Slavic, and Yiddish, warned immigrant mothers of the danger of the disease and unsanitary living, and particularly of flies, which were believed to carry the polio virus from the slums to the suburbs. Movie screens carried a slide that read "A watched child is a safe child. Swat the fly."[6]

The idea that overcrowding, poverty, and sanitary ignorance bred disease was firmly incorporated into both official and public actions. Cases that appeared in fashionable neighborhoods such as the Upper West Side were seen as anomalous and made front-page news. The illness and death of twenty-five-year-old Catherine Sefton Page, daughter-in-law of Walter Hines Page, the American ambassador to Paris, featured prominently in the *New York Times*. Page's death, according to the newspaper, "shocked the community," for "it has shown how subtle and uncontrolled are the ravages of this strange epidemic which still baffles the physicians [and] has already destroyed so many young lives."[7]

Most physicians were only able to treat polio victims with nonspecific drugs to dull pain and control fever. But the city's health laboratory also continued experiments on two polio serums begun a few years earlier by researchers at the Pasteur Institute in Paris. During the 1916 epidemic, some patients at city hospitals were given a polio virus serum cultured through horse blood, and others received a convalescent serum developed from the blood of people who had recovered from polio.[8] The popular press published sentimental stories about polio victims offering their blood for use in developing the latter serum. One man, who had a twisted leg and a limp arm, told the *New York Times*, "I've had a tough time of it. . . . Vicious people made me the butt of their fun and sensitive people have hurt me by avoiding me as if I were an unclean thing. All my life I've felt that I had no place in the world, that I was left out of everything worthwhile—until today. Now . . . I am happy because you tell me that I may be able to save some other human being from my fate. If I can do that I shall feel that I have not been wasted in this life."[9]

The 1916 epidemic occurred during a period of transition in American public health theory and practice. Through the nineteenth century, as New York City's health organizations took shape, most health reformers had based their efforts on the filth theory of disease, the idea that disease was caused by decaying materials and spread through the air by a tainted atmosphere, or "miasma." The germ theory, the notion that each case of disease was the result of a specific microorganism spread from person to person, gained support in the 1880s and 1890s. Its influence on public health work was initially limited, however, and most urban health officials continued to combat disease by searching for filth, fumigating rooms, and cleaning streets and alleyways with strong-smelling disinfectants such as chloride of lime. Although New York had some of the nation's most forward-thinking health officials in Hermann Biggs, state health commissioner, and William Hallock Park, head of the city's laboratories, even these men allowed their employees to return to traditional "antifilth" methods during the panic of the 1916 polio epidemic.

MAKING POLIO RESPECTABLE: ROOSEVELT'S EARLY EXPERIENCE, 1921–1928

During the 1920s and 1930s, middle-class children and young adults became more frequent and more visible polio victims. The experience of one of America's most famous polio sufferers, Franklin Delano Roosevelt, transformed the public perception of polio. Roosevelt's struggles with polio paralysis altered his life and his political career. In 1921, while vacationing at his family's summer home on Campobello Island off the coast of New Brunswick, Canada, Roosevelt, a young lawyer and Democratic politician from a wealthy New York family, developed the early symptoms of polio and found he was unable to move his legs.[10] Initially, his friends and political advisors denied that polio was the cause of his illness; later, even Roosevelt himself never acknowledged the seriousness of the resulting paralysis.

Eleanor Roosevelt said polio's main effect was to accentuate her husband's already great powers of self-control.[11] But the impact of paralysis on Roosevelt intrigued many observers. Some argued that his suffering transformed him, bringing out hidden compassionate qualities and drawing out compassion in others: "There can be no doubt of it, those months of pain put Franklin Roosevelt into the human race, and the permanent crippling that resulted from his disease kept him there. One no longer envied Roosevelt his head start on life."[12] Despite Roosevelt's own discounting of the impact of his paralysis, a psychologist recently argued that polio was the "central trauma" of Roosevelt's prepresidential years—a trauma that both changed him and made him President.[13] Although it is difficult to trace a direct connection, it was after the publicity about Roosevelt's illness that the public began to demonstrate a new fear of swimming pools and public baths; communities often closed them during summer months when they feared an epidemic. Roosevelt himself may have seen water as both an infecting means and a therapeutic agent, for, as he told one friend, "The water put me where I am and the water has to bring me back."[14]

Despite the strong link in the public mind between Franklin Roosevelt and polio, the New York politician's experience did not significantly alter the popular image of the handicapped. Roosevelt did not get elected to Albany as governor or to the White House as President as a disabled person. During the 1920s Roosevelt argued publicly and privately that he would walk again, and his advisors put much energy into denying the extent of his paralysis.[15] After he became President, he persuaded reporters not to describe or photograph him in his wheelchair or his leg braces. Reporters who tried to breach the unspoken ban had their cameras accidentally dropped or their film ripped out.[16]

Most Americans were not aware that their President was confined to a wheelchair, and political cartoonists often portrayed him running or jumping.[17] Roosevelt found polio to be both a political liability and an asset.[18] His political enemies used his affliction to boost rumors that he was physically, mentally, and morally unfit, and that he exploited other polio victims.[19] But in the minds of many Americans, Roosevelt, a man who had overcome physical hardship and suffering, became a powerful symbol, inspiring ordinary citizens during the Depression years. Most significantly, Roosevelt's personal experience with polio began to counter its prevailing image as an immigrant dirt disease; soon it was popularly seen as a disease that could afflict anyone, even a man from a wealthy and established family.

THE MARCH OF DIMES AND ITS EARLY TRIALS, 1927–1935

Roosevelt's interest in polio also inspired a new organization that played a major role in redefining polio: the National Foundation for Infantile Paralysis, or, as it was popularly known, the March of Dimes. The National Foundation became a central force in organizing funding for polio research and rehabilitation, and one of the largest and most successful disease philanthropies in the world. In the early 1920s Roosevelt had tried to regain his strength through water therapy at Warm Springs, a health spa in Georgia known for its water's high level of mineral salts and warm temperature. In 1924, after an Atlanta journalist reported Roosevelt's enthusiasm for the resulting improvement in his leg muscles, other paralyzed patients began to flock to Warm Springs. Roosevelt became interested in revitalizing the resort and developing polio hydrotherapy, and by 1927 had established the Warm Springs Foundation.[20]

In 1931, while Roosevelt was governor, New York State experienced another serious epidemic. Again centered in New York City, the epidemic began in early July and continued until mid-October. This time health officials confidently issued preventive warnings, and fewer families fled the epidemic's center. Reminding patients of how few children in New York's public institutions had developed paralysis in 1916, city officials called for the strict isolation of healthy children, and organizers of summer camps responded by barring parents from visiting their children during the epidemic.[21] Mayor Jimmy Walker gave the city's health commissioner, Dr. Shirley Wynne, a special appropriation of $75,000 for additional doctors and nurses. Wynne tried to calm parents by reminding them that, unlike the 1916 epidemic's 25 percent death rate, this epidemic's mortality rate was about 12 percent.[22] Wynne urged parents not to be frightened of the disease, for, with ordinary sanitary precautions, it was not very contagious, and other diseases were far more prevalent. The best means of prevention, Wynne suggested, were avoiding crowds, not swimming in polluted waters, eating only clean, wholesome food, disposing of all house vermin and insects, and washing all eating utensils. City officials also continued their use of convalescent blood serum as a preventive, and in early August Governor Roosevelt contributed a pint of his blood.[23]

Other actions suggest that the medical profession and the public remained uncertain of the way polio spread or how to prevent it. The city engaged in a fervent sanitary drive, and the city's magistrates were asked to cooperate fully, particularly regarding health violations by soda fountains and restaurants. At meetings at Wynne's office, city physicians debated the role of healthy carriers and the possibility of an intermediate host such as a rat, mouse, or fly.[24] There was a lingering fear that objects as well as people could carry the disease. The head of the Department of Sanitation volunteered the use of five trucks "to remove personal property of victims of disease." Wynne accepted this offer, explaining that "it was an extra precaution . . . although there was little danger of contagion from bedclothing or personal belongings."[25] A popular fear of water appeared in the public concern over the possible danger of public beaches, but health officials were unsure whether water played a significant role in the spread of polio. In August, Lincoln Park officials banned all swimming at public beaches, but after a mass protest meeting the local board of health relented and lifted the ban.[26]

Clearly, the public was not ready to accept overstringent hygienic advice. City medical examiner Dr. John Oberwager warned parents at a meeting in Brooklyn, "Don't ever kiss your children or allow them to be kissed, now or at any other time. . . . It is a legal, moral, parental duty. A kiss is the easiest way of spreading disease." But, according to a *New York Times* report, his listeners' response was not enthusiastic. "A hum of surprise, tinged with disapproval, rose from the audience."[27]

A series of polio epidemics throughout the United States during the 1930s raised public awareness of polio aftercare as a national problem. New York philanthropists established an Infantile Paralysis Commission to raise money for physical therapy, surgery, and orthopedic supplies. By this time polio had become seen as "Roosevelt's disease." After New York's governor was elected President in 1932, a public relations firm suggested to the commission that it raise money for polio patients across the country by holding ballroom dances on Roosevelt's birthday. Participants were exhorted to "dance so that others may walk." The first set of Birthday Balls in January 1934 raised $1 million, the second $1.25 million.[28]

These campaigns established the themes of later polio fund-raising. They had no formal link to the government or scientific agencies. They were organized at both the local and national level, and they relied largely on volunteer work. Most campaigns were directed by philanthropic businessmen, not doctors or scientists. They were advanced by sophisticated advertising techniques, oriented around children as both potential victims and donors. And, most significantly, they promoted the idea of polio as a danger to all. As the crippled young girl on the March of Dimes 1942 billboard announced, "I could be *your* child."[29]

In September 1937, Roosevelt announced the establishment of the National Foundation for Infantile Paralysis, a national nonprofit organization distinct from his Warm Springs Foundation. In November, during a Hollywood fundraiser, Eddie Cantor, a radio and vaudeville entertainer, suggested that radio stations asking listeners to send money to the White House call the campaign the March of Dimes.[30] With its headquarters in New York City, the National Foundation solidified the increasingly respectable image of the disease and turned the funding of polio treatment and research into a mass-marketing enterprise in which scientists no longer played a determining role. Its massive funding of scientific research in an era with few other large funding agencies for medical science altered the direction of polio research and spurred the rise of a new generation of virologists who came to see viruses as distinct from bacteria and concentrated much of their research around the polio virus.

The National Foundation's campaign techniques were unashamedly sentimental, going far beyond the efforts of the American Heart Association, the American Cancer Society, or the National Tuberculosis Association. The National Foundation's popular *Infantile Paralysis* magazine portrayed polio as an agent of "malevolence." "Each year it makes its awful visitations. Each year it seeks to maim and cripple our helpless babes, our happy youths, and, in some instances, those in maturity."[31] Such campaigns exploited the emotional pull of crippled children, and March of Dimes cans and posters usually featured a child on crutches. "The spectacle of a brave but paralyzed little child, boldly attempting his first steps with ·steel braces attached to his legs, was well-nigh irresistible," a polio researcher later commented.[32]

As public awareness and fears of polio grew, the National Foundation recast the conquest of the disease as a kind of holy quest. Most American scientists were uneasy about the National Foundation's upbeat promises of children learning to walk and researchers finding a polio cure. They saw the National Foundation as "sudden appearance of a fairy godmother of quite mammoth proportions who thrived on publicity."[33] Their greatest unease probably derived from the fact that the directors of the National Foundation were not scientists but laymen. Not surprisingly, the National Foundation was caught up in the territorial and professional battles within the scientific community, particularly those between older bacteriologists and the new generation of virologists.

POLIO VIROLOGY AND THERAPY, 1935–1950

The National Foundation contributed significantly to the development of the discipline of virology in the United States. In fact, for American scientists, investigating the nature of the polio virus came to epitomize viral research. Potential grantees quickly learned to phrase their proposals so as to link them to part of the National Foundation's polio research agenda.

At the same time, the epidemiological picture of polio was shifting. After researchers discovered high levels of the virus in the sewage systems of urban areas such as Manhattan and New Haven, they began to argue that the infection was widespread. Further, they suggested that polio was not primarily a disease of the central nervous system, but a general systemic infection centered in the intestines. Polio epidemics appeared once every two or three years as previously exposed groups became infected by more than one type of polio virus. Clean, protected middle-class children tended to have lower levels of polio antibodies than poor urban children. Consequently, adequate sanitation might not be as preventive as health officials had assumed. Polio, in fact, might be a disease of cleanliness rather than dirt.

During the 1930s and 1940s, other earlier scientific tenets about the nature of polio were also undermined. The Rockefeller Institute's model of polio had proposed that the polio virus entered the body through the nose and traveled directly to the brain and spinal cord along nerve pathways. This model boded ill for the development of a polio vaccine, for it was accepted that any vaccine grown from nerve cells could cause brain infections such as encephalitis.[34] In 1935 the National Foundation funded the trials of an experimental polio vaccine that had been developed by New York City researchers. The New York trials were a disaster: some vaccinated children were paralyzed, and the results turned many physicians in the 1930s away from the idea of a vaccine.[35] By the 1940s, however, scientists had come to believe that the polio virus only occasionally attacked the nerve tissues. As young virologists developed ways to grow the virus outside neural tissues, they raised new hopes for the possibility of a safe vaccine. The most significant tissue culture work was conducted by John Enders, Thomas Weller, and Frederick Robbins at a newly established infectious disease laboratory at the Children's Hospital in Boston. In 1948, under a National Foundation grant, Enders's team was able to cultivate a strain of the polio virus in non-neurological tissue. The discovery of new properties of the polio virus, along with ways to assess the appearance of the virus in tissue culture rather than through laboratory animals, cleared the way for safe vaccine production and won the team the Nobel Prize in 1954.[36]

This era also saw new approaches to polio therapy. In the 1930s the National Foundation began funding Drinker respirators, or iron lung machines, which were first used in 1929 to help paralyzed patients breathe.[37] In 1940 Elizabeth Kenny, a charismatic nurse, arrived in the United States from Australia, armed with a new therapy for training paralyzed muscles. Although initially hesitant, the National Foundation began to provide funding to train Kenny therapists after doctors at the University of Minnesota publicized her impressive results. Kenny rejected the prevailing emphasis on splints and limited muscle movement for paralyzed patients. Instead, she urged the use of heat and the active training of muscles. The skepticism of the established medical profession about Kenny's concept of polio as a disease that affected the muscles and skin but not nerves put the National Foundation in a difficult position, and within a few years the National Foundation, although it continued to fund the training of Kenny therapists, had halted its public support of Kenny herself.[38] Kenny's own foundation, established in 1943, became the only private grant agency that opposed National Foundation policy during this period.[39]

When New York City experienced another serious polio epidemic, in 1949, the public turned for advice to the National Foundation. The tumultuous state of polio research was reflected in the organization's somewhat defensive response. In August 1949, Harry Weaver, the new director of research, announced from the National Foundation's headquarters at 120 Broadway that many popular notions about how polio was contracted and spread were "without scientific basis." Weaver explained that the epidemic would not be halted by closing schools, churches, parks, or other gathering places, or by the use of insect spray. There was no evidence that children got polio from swimming in beaches or pools, although, Weaver warned, the concentration of people in such places and sudden chilling after bathing might give the infection a good chance to develop. Polio was usually spread through intimate physical contact, he explained, within households and families but not on streets or in theaters. Those who developed paralytic symptoms were probably vulnerable as the result of heredity and environmental factors that scientists did not thoroughly understand. Nor was it true that medical science knew "absolutely nothing" about the disease, for the National Foundation had been spending $2 million a year on research.[40] Later in August an article in *Time* magazine suggested that the National Foundation's leadership was tinged in the public mind with hyperbole. *Time* commented on the way the National Foundation's campaigns played on parents' heartstrings, arguing that parents could scarcely think of polio without panic.[41]

By August 20, 1949, New York City had the highest number of polio cases ever reported in one week: 3,442.[42] Trying to dampen public concern, city health officials reminded the public that most people with polio recovered, only 15 percent were left handicapped, and the death rate was usually less than 10 percent.[43] Despite the National Foundation's slogan that "facts fight fears," city officials admitted that medical scientists still did not know how to prevent or cure the disease.[44]

The 1949 epidemic also illuminated the extent to which aspects of polio's epidemiology had become part of public expectations. Some enterprising citizens had come to depend on one polio epidemic protecting a population from a second outbreak. After a serious epidemic in 1948, the Continental Casualty Company of Chicago had offered the public polio insurance for up to $5,000.

The company sold more than 500,000 policies. After the 1949 epidemic it faced a raft of claims. The vice-president admitted that the company would "lose plenty" but claimed that it had not intended to do more than break even, for "we didn't feel it would be good policy to make scads of money out of something as dreadful as polio."[45]

NEW HORIZONS: THE POLIO VACCINES, 1950–1990

By 1950 the term *polio* had become accepted for both the disease and its victims. As one popular writer reflected, "*polio*—the new name you get after Infantile Paralysis slugs you. Forever after you will be known as a *polio*."[46] As the disease began to affect older children and adults, a new genre of polio literature appeared: the reminiscences of adult polio victims. Sometimes maudlin, often sentimental, and usually optimistic, these works dealt with the daily domestic struggles and achievements of handicapped adults, their reliance on therapists and machines, and their hope that science would find a polio cure.[47]

After World War II, polio became an interdisciplinary scientific problem. The National Foundation initiated a major research effort led by Harry Weaver, who encouraged researchers to come together in a series of conferences "engineered in such a way that the independent-minded scientists would not know they were being directed."[48] In the 1930s and 1940s, the National Foundation had funded polio research on broad topics including the role of nutrition for polio prevention and possible chemical cures.[49] But as Weaver adopted the view of younger virologists, he became increasingly antagonistic to the idea of polio as a neurotropic virus and more hopeful about the possibility of a polio vaccine. By the early 1950s the National Foundation had begun to encourage the funding of work in virological pathology and immunology and to popularize the hope for a polio vaccine. "Instead of waiting to heal the ravages of polio after it strikes, we must boldly try to prevent it," polio fund-raisers were urged to tell lay audiences in 1954. The price of success was high, but "it is a new conception that is nation-wide in scope, worldwide in implications, and limitless in its promise of new horizons in the realm of public health." The victory over polio was, the National Foundation proclaimed, "the exciting culmination of a unique partnership between men and science and millions of ordinary people—joined together voluntarily under the banner of the National Foundation."[50]

As scientists began to develop polio vaccines, the National Foundation became embroiled in major disagreements among virologists over immunological theory and practice. Particularly at issue were the relative safety and efficacy of a live-virus vaccine, based on classic immunological principles, as opposed to a killed-virus vaccine.[51] Jonas Salk believed that a killed-virus vaccine could induce effective immunity, but Albert Sabin, John Enders, and others argued that only a live-virus vaccine would raise antibody levels high enough to produce lasting immunity.

Salk had arrived at the University of Pittsburgh in 1947, seeking independence and distance from the anti-Semitism that had hindered him from pursuing his career in more prestigious New York laboratories. The son of a Jewish garment manufacturer, Salk had graduated from New York's City College and received a medical degree from New York University's College of Medicine. While he was funded by the National Foundation in Pittsburgh, Salk, using Enders's new tissue-culture methods, developed a killed-virus polio vaccine that he initially tested on himself, his family, and a group of handicapped children.[52] In 1953 Salk and the National Foundation decided to organize national trials to test his vaccine. Their decision horrified more conservative members of the scientific establishment, including Albert Sabin, who challenged the validity of a killed-virus vaccine. Sabin, like Salk, was the son of immigrants, and he had also graduated from New York University's College of Medicine. He had worked at the Rockefeller Institute but had left to pursue his own studies of polio; in the 1950s he developed a live-virus polio vaccine that he tested on himself, his family, and two hundred federal prisoners. By then the National Foundation was committed to supporting Salk's vaccine, so, in 1957, in a move unusual in the Cold War years, Sabin conducted his massive trials in the Soviet Union.[53]

The Salk vaccine trials suffered from a number of professional and political troubles: disagreements over the kind of control groups, the resignation of Harry Weaver, the caution of the National Institutes of Health, and the difficulty of choosing an objective assessor of the trial results. Medical journalist and muckraker Paul de Kruif—who had formerly worked briefly as a bacteriologist at the Rockefeller Institute—contributed to the general unease by advising newspaper columnist Walter Winchell two weeks before the trials to tell the public about the problems pharmaceutical laboratories had encountered in developing mass-production techniques for the vaccine. Partly as a result of this adverse publicity, approximately eighteen thousand children dropped out of the trials. Nonetheless, from April to June 1954, 1.8 million children between the ages of six and nine were vaccinated in forty-four states.[54] On April 12, 1955, epidemiologist Thomas Francis presented his report at an open meeting organized by the National Foundation. The date, the tenth anniversary of Roosevelt's death, was simply coincidental according to National Foundation officials. Francis tried to limit sensationalism but conceded that the vaccine had been largely effective: it had protected 60 to 70 percent from the Type I Virus, 60 percent from spinal paralysis, and, most encouragingly, over 90 percent from the most debilitating kind of polio, bulbar (or respiratory) paralysis. In his own speech at the meeting, however, Salk claimed that his new methods of vaccine preparation had eliminated any problems, making his killed-virus vaccine 100 percent effective. Salk's comment angered

Francis and other cautious scientists, who were already wary of Salk's partici-
pation in the National Foundation's publicity campaigns. Among many of his
colleagues, Salk was perceived as a publicity seeker, and the National Foundation's overwhelming support of his killed-virus vaccine only exacerbated
relations within the virological community.[55] Nevertheless, the vaccine was
approved the same day and immediately licensed by federal officials.[56]

Both Salk's and the National Foundation's reputations were tarnished by
what became known as the Cutter incident. Within fifteen days of Francis's
1955 report, cases of paralysis were reported among children who had received the vaccine. After federal officials from the Communicable Disease
Center established that these cases were the result of a defective batch of
vaccine prepared by the Cutter Laboratories of Berkeley, California, Surgeon
General Leonard Scheele halted the vaccination program for a week. By mid-
summer 1955, Scheele established a new Polio Surveillance Unit and tightened vaccine testing requirements. Altogether, 204 cases, including 11 deaths,
were linked to the Salk vaccine, and 40 suits for damages were later settled in
California courts.[57] Virologists initiated an investigation to determine whether
the diaster was the result of improper laboratory methods or whether something in Salk's procedures had led to the appearance of live virus in the vaccine. The issue still remains unresolved. During meetings in June 1955,
scientific experts voted eight to three to continue the vaccination program, but
they later agreed that Salk must find a substitute for the strong Mahoney Type
I strain he had used. A few virologists, including John Enders, also attacked
Salk's inactivation "margins of safety" theory. Scheele's final report led to the
resignation of Eisenhower's Secretary for Health, Education, and Welfare,
Oveta Culp Hobby, and a year later, of Scheele himself.[58]

The development of a live-virus vaccine did not proceed smoothly either.
Virologists Herald Cox and Hilary Koprowski, for example, developed a live-
virus vaccine at the Lederle laboratories of the American Cyanamid Company. In 1950 they tested the vaccine on a group of mentally handicapped
children at the New York state institution.[59] Although critics questioned the
ethics of calling these children "volunteers" and pointed out the possibility
that the attenuated virus had reverted to virulence in vaccinated children's
stools, both men continued, separately, to test their vaccines in Northern Ireland and the former Belgian Congo. Their vaccines began to lose popularity
after vaccine-linked polio cases were reported in Northern Ireland, however,
and organizers in Africa came in conflict with policies of the World Health
Organization.[60]

Albert Sabin played a major role in attacking the Salk vaccine, and at times
the polio story became a public fight between the two eminent Jewish scientists from New York.[61] In 1960 Sabin announced that his live-virus had been
successfully tested on over 4.5 million people in the U.S.S.R., Singapore, and
Mexico.[62] Sabin received international acclaim, but United States federal offi-

cials still hesitated to license a live-virus vaccine. In 1960, the Lederle-Cox vaccine struck further disaster when cases resulting in paralysis occurred after trials in Dade County (Florida) and in West Germany.[63] There were also disturbing reports of increased numbers of polio cases in communities vaccinated with the Salk vaccine. Salk explained these cases as the result of the public's failure to take the right number of vaccine injections, an argument that seemed to reinforce the appeal of Sabin's easy-to-take syrup.[64] In 1961 the Surgeon General licensed the Sabin vaccine (and later the Lederle-Cox and Koprowski vaccines), but this time there were few public demonstrations. "The people had grown weary of polio heroes," a commentator later reflected.[65]

The Sabin vaccine also encountered production problems, although there was no single Cutter-like incident. In 1962 the first reports of Sabin-vaccine-associated paralysis appeared in the United States. The cases were not just among the vaccinated but also among children and adults who had become infected through the stools of vaccinated children as the attenuated virus had mutated into a more virulent strain. Although detective novelist Alistair Mac-Lean exaggerated when he described the invention of a mutated polio virus in *The Satan Bug* (1962) as "the most terrible and terrifying weapon mankind has ever known," health officials acknowledged that a live-virus vaccine did pose some risk.[66] By 1964 there was a new federal polio vaccine policy based on the acceptance of some risk; officials suggested that first only those under eighteen and later only infants and preschool children should receive the oral live-virus vaccine. This new approach involved instituting a reeducation program for the public in order to reverse the National Foundation's effective campaign, which had urged every American, young and old, to be vaccinated with the Salk vaccine.[67] Certainly the image of polio and its public health prevention had markedly changed since the disease was first associated with New York City slums and prevention with cleaning the homes and streets of the immigrant poor.

POLIO IN PERSPECTIVE

The 1950s and 1960s are considered the pinnacle moment in the polio story. Despite the Cutter incident, the Salk and Sabin vaccines reinforced popular faith in the power of science. Medical speakers today still refer to the victory over polio as an example of the lifesaving potential of science in medicine.

The massive publicity over the Salk vaccine trials, however, raised tensions in the scientific community over the ways the media turned a scientist into a hero. When Enders and his team, but not Jonas Salk, were honored with the Nobel Prize, the scientific community saw the choice as a comment on both Salk's role in the vaccine trials and the National Foundation's unabashed campaigning. The National Foundation remains an important health-funding organization today, its headquarters now in White Plains, New York, but with the expansion of federal research funding and other private health agencies, it is no longer as prestigious or influential as in its earlier years. In 1958 the directors of the National Foundation reoriented the March of Dimes campaigns away from polio to other health problems, such as arthritis and birth defects.[68]

In the last decade, with the surprising appearance of muscle weakness among older polio victims (a condition called postpolio syndrome), polio has been "rediscovered" by both scientists and the public. And with the AIDS epidemic, issues relating to the nature and control of infectious diseases have again caught the public imagination. AIDS has raised ethical and health policy issues strikingly similar to those of the past. The popular and official interest in AIDS prevention and treatment has developed as AIDS is seen to threaten not only gay bars and drug-ridden housing projects but also the homes and schools of middle-class heterosexual Americans—just as the expansion of public funding for and interest in polio came with the transformation of polio's image from an immigrant dirt disease to "Roosevelt's disease."

The history of polio leads us from a fear of immigrants as the carriers of an insidious dirt disease to national accolades for two scientists from Jewish immigrant families who developed vaccines to prevent a disease believed to endanger all members of the community. Jonas Salk, now an established virological statesman, has spoken encouragingly of the similarities between the polio and AIDS viruses in the search for a vaccine. But as New York City's experiences with polio suggest, control and victory over a disease are fraught with prejudice and politics.

Notes

My thanks for their support and editorial comments to Maureen Dyer, June Factor, Sue Lederer, and John Harley Warner.

1. William Harvey Young to Blanche DeBra Young, July 6, 1916. Letters in possession of James Harvey Young, Decatur, Georgia.

2. Haven Emerson, *A Monograph on the Epidemic of Poliomyelitis (Infantile Paralysis) in New York City in 1916: Based on the Official Reports of the Bureaus of the Department of Health* (New York: Department of Health, 1917); see also Naomi Rogers, *Dirt and Disease: Polio before FDR* (New Brunswick, N.J.: Rutgers University Press, 1992). New York State had over thirteen thousand cases, New Jersey more than two thousand, and many other states reported cases into the hundreds.

3. *New York Times*, July 8, 1916.

4. *Newark Evening News*, July 19, 1916.

5. *Newark Evening News*, July 12, 1916.

6. *New York Times*, July 9, 1916; *Philadelphia Evening Bulletin*, July 6, 1916; and see also Naomi Rogers, "Germs with Legs: Flies, Disease and the New Public Health," *Bulletin of the History of Medicine* 64 (1989): 509–539.

7. *New York Times*, August 14, 1916.

8. Emerson, *Monograph*, 246.

9. *New York Times*, August 9, 1916.

10. See Finis Farr, *FDR* (New Rochelle, N.Y.: Arlington House, 172), 128–130. See also Hugh Gregory Gallagher, *FDR's Splendid Deception* (New York: Dodd, Mead, 1988), and Richard Thayer Goldberg, *The Making of Franklin D. Roosevelt: Triumph over Disability* (Cambridge, Mass.: Abt Books, 1981).

11. Frank Freidel, *Franklin D. Roosevelt: The Ordeal* (Boston: Little, Brown, 1954), 121.

12. Farr, *FDR*, 132.

13. Goldberg, *The Making of Roosevelt*, vii–viii.

14. Freidel, *Ordeal*, 113.

15. Gallagher, *Deception*, 18, 78; Goldberg, *The Making of Roosevelt*, 131.

16. Gallagher, *Deception*, 93–94, 163.

17. Ibid., 210–213.

18. Goldberg, *The Making of Roosevelt*, 170.

19. Ibid., 171; Gallagher, *Deception*, 85, 147; Farr, *FDR*, 144–145.

20. Goldberg, *The Making of Roosevelt*, 75–76.

21. *New York Times*, August 8, 1931.

22. *New York Times*, August 4, 1931.

23. *New York Times*, August 6, 1931.

24. *New York Times*, August 6, 1931.

25. *New York Times*, August 7, 1931.

26. *New York Times*, August 8, 1931.

27. *New York Times*, August 6, 1931.

28. Aaron E. Klein, *Trial by Fury: The Polio Vaccine Controversy* (New York: Charles Scribner's Sons, 1972), 151–156. See also Jane S. Smith, *Patenting the Sun: Polio and the Salk Vaccine* (New York: William Morrow, 1990).

29. Photograph in Foster and Kleiser Scrapbook, 1942, Polio Collection, file group 3130, Franklin D. Roosevelt Library, Hyde Park, New York.

30. Klein, *Trial by Fury*, 17; see also Roland Berg, *Polio and Its Problems* (Philadelphia: J. B. Lippincott, 1948).

31. Keith Morgan, *The Star Contest on the American Flag: An Address Delivered to the Nation over the Mutual Broadcasting System* (New York: Privately printed, 1940), [17]. See also *Infantile Paralysis Magazine* (1939) [1].

32. John R. Paul, *A History of Poliomyelitis* (New Haven: Yale University Press, 1971), 304.

33. Ibid., 311.

34. Paul de Kruif, *The Fight for Life* (New York: Harcourt, Brace, 1938), 154.

35. Paul de Kruif, *The Sweeping Wind: A Memoir* (New York: Harcourt, Brace and World, 1962), 178–179. See also Richard Carter, *Breakthrough: The Saga of Jonas Salk* (New York: Trident Press, 1966).

36. Paul, *History*, 374–381.

37. Paul, *History*, 330–333.

38. Berg, *Polio and Its Problems*, 125–126; see also Victor Cohn, *Sister Kenny: The Woman Who Challenged the Doctors* (Minneapolis: University of Minnesota, 1975).

39. Paul, *History*, 340–345.

40. *New York Times*, August 9, 1949.

41. *Time*, August 22, 1949.

42. *New York Times*, August 26, 1949.

43. *New York Times*, August 7, 1949.

44. *New York Times*, August 7, 1949.

45. *Newsweek*, September 5, 1949.

46. Turnley Walker, *Rise Up and Walk* (New York: E. P. Dutton, 1950), 7.

47. See, for example, Walker, *Rise Up and Walk*; Milton Lomask, *The Man in the Iron Lung: The Frederick B. Snite, Jr., Story* (Garden City, N.Y.: Doubleday, 1956); and Anne Walers and Jim Marugg, *Beyond Endurance* (New York: Harper and Brothers, 1954).

48. Klein, *Trial by Fury*, 46.

49. Berg, *Polio and Its Problems*, 63–77, 108–110.

50. National Foundation for Infantile Paralysis, *1954 Speakers Handbook* (New York: Public Relations Department, National Foundation, [1954]), 3–5.

51. Smith, *Patenting the Sun*, 146–149.

52. Ibid., 103–106, 137–139, 147–148.

53. Klein, *Trial by Fury*, 140–141; Paul, *History*, 445–448, 455–459.

54. Paul, *History*, 422–428.

55. Ibid., 423–424, 443–444; see also Klein, *Trial by Fury*.

56. See Naomi Rogers, "Thomas Francis, Jr.: From the Bench to the Field," in Joel Howell, ed., *Medical Lives and Scientific Medicine at Michigan, 1861–1969* (Ann Arbor: University of Michigan Press, 1993), 161–187.

57. Smith, *Patenting the Sun*, 364–367.

58. Ibid.

59. Carter, *Breakthrough*, 109–111; see also Klein, *Trial by Fury*.

60. Klein, *Trial by Fury*, 135–136, 140–141.

61. Carter, *Breakthrough*, 81–82, 111–117.

62. Paul, *History*, 455–459.

63. Klein, *Trial by Fury*, 142–147; see also Paul, *History*.

64. Klein, *Trial by Fury*, 146.

65. Ibid., 147.

66. Alistair MacLean, *The Satan Bug* (Greenwich, Conn.: Fawcett, 1962), 42.

67. Paul, *History*, 465–467.

68. Smith, *Patenting the Sun*, 72–73.

RONALD BAYER

The Dependent Center: The First Decade of the AIDS Epidemic in New York City

Epidemics are by their nature both biological and political events. Just as a new microparasitic threat may destabilize the biological status quo, the rapid increase in disease may pose challenges to the political system. Much depends on the intensity of the epidemic threat, the severity of its exactions, the breadth of its assault, its impact on cultural and social institutions and values, and the social standing of those who are affected. Inevitably, the responses provoked by an epidemic challenge will reflect prevailing social arrangements. Those very responses will in turn shape a society's experience of the biological threat.

Insights about the impact of epidemic disease on society—the lessons of Charles Rosenberg's *Cholera Years* that appeared in 1962 and William McNeill's *Plagues and People*, published fourteen years later—took on an unanticipated immediacy in 1981, when the AIDS epidemic was first publicly recognized.

EPIDEMIOLOGY AND THE SOCIAL DIMENSIONS OF THE EPIDEMIC

What began with reports in mid-1981 of unusual and lethal diseases among gay men on both the East and West coasts has developed into an epidemic with profound impact in the United States. Also in 1981, reports of disease began to appear in Africa and Haiti, presaging the worldwide pandemic of AIDS. The United States would emerge as the center of the epidemic that was taking shape in the economically developed world, as East Africa would in the Third World. New York City was destined to become the epicenter of the American epidemic.

It was in June 1981 that the Centers for Disease Control (CDC) reported that between October 1980 and May 1981 five young men had been diagnosed with *pneumocystis carinii* pneumonia (PCP). All were gay.[1] One month later the CDC reported that in the prior thirty months, 26 cases of an unusual malignancy, Kaposi's sarcoma (KS), had been diagnosed in New York City and California. They, too, were among gay men.[2] On the first anniversary of the

CDC's first report, the federal agency announced that 355 cases of disease had been reported. Eighty percent involved gay or bisexual men. Among the heterosexuals, the most striking characteristic was a history of intravenous drug use. Ultimately PCP, KS, and a host of other disorders were linked to the assault on the immune systems that each of those who had fallen ill had experienced, and the epidemic was given the name by which it would be known, AIDS (Acquired Immune Deficiency Syndrome).

Only after the Human Immunodeficiency Virus (HIV), the etiological agent responsible for AIDS, was identified, in 1984, and when a diagnostic test was developed to detect its presence, in 1985, was it possible to speak of the dimensions and history of the epidemic with any accuracy. The first manifestations of disease recorded by the CDC had been but the end stages of hidden infections that had occurred years earlier.

In New York City, retrospective analyses of medical records detected the first cases of AIDS in children in 1977. Their mothers, therefore, must have been infected prior to that time.[3] A study of one cohort of drug users in Manhattan found that as of 1978, 9 percent were already infected with HIV. By 1980, a year before the first official reports of AIDS, 38 percent were infected.[4]

At the end of the epidemic's first decade, widely accepted estimates suggested that as many as 200,000 New Yorkers were infected with the AIDS virus.[5] As of June, 1992, 41,598 cases had been reported (949 of which were among children); 28,871 people were dead. Gay and bisexual men bore the brunt of the epidemic in the first years. By 1992, however, what had once been called the "gay plague" was increasingly a disease of poor drug users and their sexual partners. Sixty-four percent of those who had been diagnosed were black and Hispanic.[6] Although no dimension of the city's social, cultural, or political life remained unaffected by the epidemic, the communities within which those most at risk for HIV lived were most profoundly touched. The West Village and other locales where gay men lived in great concentrations, Harlem, the South Bronx, and parts of Brooklyn where intravenous drug use was so prevalent were severely touched. Among gay men entire friendship networks became sick and succumbed. Among blacks and Hispanics entire families—mothers, fathers, and their children—fell ill and died. Grandmothers were often left to care for those children who were orphaned, while other children were relegated to New York City's inadequate foster care system.

One study estimated that between 9 and 21 percent of all males between twenty-five and forty-four years of age were infected with HIV in the South Bronx.[7] A survey of infection among women in New York State who had given birth in 1988 underscored the differential impact of the epidemic. The prevalence of HIV infection outside New York City was .16 percent (1 in 643). In Queens the rate was .68 percent, in Brooklyn 1.25 percent, in Manhattan 1.69 percent, and in the Bronx the figure was 1.89 percent (1 in 53). Two percent of black women who had given birth and 1.66 percent of the Hispanic women who had done so were infected with the AIDS virus.[8] As a consequence of this pattern of infection, 90 percent of pediatric AIDS cases in New York were black or Hispanic.[9]

Although initial uncertainty about the mechanisms through which AIDS could be transmitted provoked considerable anxiety about the risks of casual transmission, epidemiological and scientific study rapidly defined the limited routes of transmission. Against public anxiety, public health officials sought to provide the antidote of reassurance. HIV was spread by sexual intercourse; by sharing drug-injection equipment contaminated with infected blood; from mother to fetus; by infected blood transfusions; and in rare cases by blood contact between patients and health care workers. There were no other risks of contagion. Recent immigrants from Haiti were initially designated a special risk group because of an apparently elevated prevalence of AIDS among such men and women in New York, as well as because of the striking dimensions of the epidemic in Haiti itself. Closer analysis of the epidemiological data, in addition to political concerns over stigmatization, led New York City's health authorities to end the public designation of Haitians as a separate risk category. In the end, sexual orientation, the social demography of intravenous drug use, and the lines of social cleavage that affect the likelihood of sexual contact across class and ethnic lines would serve to define the epidemic's course in the city.

As a sudden threat, one for which there was no effective medical response, AIDS posed a challenge to the communities most affected, to the public health system that would be called upon to contain the epidemic's spread, and to the political system that would have to mobilize both the necessary material sources to fund such an effort and the leadership necessary to preserve public calm in the face of anxiety. There were, however, limits to what the city could do. Decisions about resources for care and prevention that would affect the capacity of the municipal authorities to respond to AIDS were often made in Albany and Washington, D.C. At the center of the epidemic, New York was, nevertheless, in an utterly dependent position.

FIRST RESPONSES: 1981–1985

Awareness of the threatening new afflictions besetting gay men preceded any definitive understanding of what it was that had caused the life-threatening disease. Why were gay men at risk? Had a pathogen that was sexually transmitted entered the gay community? Was there something unique to the pattern of sexual behavior among urban gay men that subverted the body's disease-fighting capacity?

The tentative manner in which the gay community first addressed the issue of the potential sexual transmission of AIDS in 1981 and 1982 reflected both profound disagreements and deep anxieties about how the open discussion of gay sexual culture and practices might create an ideological climate within which the hard-won advances of greater sexual tolerance in America could be swept away in the name of public health. Writing about these two dimensions of the debate in the *Native*, New York's gay newspaper, Dr. Lawrence Mass said, "Outside the gay community the current epidemic is already inspiring the kind of medical-moral speculation that swept England a century ago. Within the gay community, a parallel crisis of ideology is threatening to explode. With much confusion on all sides, advocates of sexual 'fulfillment' are being opposed to critics of 'promiscuity.'"[10]

Nevertheless, as gay men spoke and wrote about AIDS there began to emerge a consensus about what needed to be done. By mid-1982 the voice of sexual moderation began to assume the characteristics of an orthodoxy demanded by health, the health of each gay man as well as the health of the gay community. Physicians, many of them gay, began to urge their patients to exercise caution, to choose fewer partners, those in good health. "It is not sex itself as the moralists would have it, but the number of different sexual encounters that may increase risk."[11]

But the brutal truth of the consensus on the risks of sexual encounters with many anonymous partners—which had come to define the cultural norm of some parts of the gay community—did in fact provoke expressions of opposition, some that reflected the desperation of those who believed their newfound freedoms were under attack. The calls for restraint were sometimes seen as nothing more than thinly disguised demands for a return to sexual conventionality. Once again, it was argued, physicians were seeking to establish their dominance over homosexuality, now with the collaboration of those who carried their message in the gay press.[12]

Writing in response to the cautionary advice that appeared in the *Native,* one correspondent asserted that the risks involved in hailing a taxi were a greater threat than sexual relations with a stranger. Faced with constraints that would follow from the warnings about promiscuity—"they are actually asking us to avoid all casual sex"—he preferred to take his chances. "I refuse to blight my life in order—supposedly—to preserve it."[13]

Such resistance drew the response of Larry Kramer, the playwright and AIDS activist, in "1,112 and Counting," a dramatic call to arms published in the *Native* in 1983. Like his earlier appeals to the gay community, this article thundered its message of alarm. "Our continued existence as gay men upon the face of this earth is at stake. Unless we fight for our lives, we shall die. In all the history of homosexuality, we have never been so close to death and extinction before. Many of us are dying and are dead already." A demand for more money for research into AIDS and a denunciation of government officials who failed to respond because it was the lives of gay men that were at stake, this jeremiad also pointed a finger of accusation at gay men who refused to change their sexual lives. "I am sick of guys who moan that giving up careless sex until this blows over is worse than death. How can they value life so little and cocks and asses so much? Come with me, guys, while I visit a few of our friends in intensive care. . . . Notice the looks in their eyes, guys. They'd give up sex forever if you could promise them life."[14]

Unlike the situation that existed in San Francisco, where a politically well organized gay community was able to press local officials to launch campaigns designed to alert gay men to the threat of AIDS, New York's public health officials moved much more slowly.[15] In the face of such an institutional vacuum, the Gay Men's Health Crisis (GMHC) was formed in 1982. As a voluntary association devoted to education and service, it would ultimately serve as a model of communal self-help efforts in both the United States and Europe. With its origins in the white middle-class gay community, it was inevitable that the GMHC's largely volunteer staff would, especially in the first years of the epidemic, primarily serve such men.

There was little to compare with such efforts in the black and Hispanic communities. Limited resources, the perception of AIDS as a disease of white gay men, homophobia, and profound antagonism to the drug users with whom so much of the terror of ghetto life was linked all conspired to produce virtual silence on the issue of AIDS.[16] Writing as late as 1987, Sam Friedman could note, "There has been little organized Black or Hispanic response. The major Black and Hispanic institutions have done little or nothing, and there has been no grass roots flowering of AIDS-related organizations."[17] That was to change in the last years of the 1980s, but by then years of HIV transmission had already sown the seeds of a grave public health crisis.

The New York City Department of Health responded with extraordinary caution to the emerging challenge in the early 1980s. Having emerged from the fiscal crisis of the 1970s with a weakened professional staff and a loss of its former prestige, it was, nevertheless, afforded the opportunity to assume a leadership role under the direction of Commissioner David Sencer, former director of the Centers for Disease Control. Although the Department of Health had responsibility neither for the provision of health care to the poor—that was the task of the Health and Hospitals Corporation—nor for the provision of drug abuse services—that was a responsibility of the state's Department of Substance Abuse Services—the department could have assumed a critical role in mobilizing public support for a campaign against AIDS and for providing social and clinical services to those who were ill. It did not. Characteristically, in calling a meeting of all interested parties in the city to discuss AIDS, the department declared that it sought "not to direct but to provide a neutral meeting ground."[18]

Sencer, who had presided over the swine flu vaccine fiasco while at the CDC, an effort to mobilize the nation for mass vaccination against an epidemic that never materialized, was wary of launching another dramatic effort.[19] He was not convinced, at least initially, that AIDS would pose a grave threat.

Finally, as public anxiety began to mount, he believed that the assumption of a relatively low profile would contribute to the creation of a climate within which rash acts of discrimination against those with AIDS, and within which calls for repressive measures in the name of public health would be less likely to occur.

In assuming such a posture, he fashioned policies that often coincided with those being pressed by the gay community, which was increasingly concerned about how the threat of AIDS might contribute to the subversion of the hard-won rights of sexual privacy. Indeed, Sencer's recognition that overcoming the deep fear and suspicion that gay men had of agencies of the state was critical to any public health effort to control AIDS was a central element in shaping his initiatives. If the goal of AIDS-prevention policy was to foster the modification of behaviors linked to the spread of disease, then no effort that would create a breach between those at risk for infection and the authorities would advance the public health. In assuming such a stance, much of the traditional repertoire of the response to epidemic threats had to be subject to reconsideration. To those who viewed Sencer's perspective—shared to some degree by many public health officials in cities and states confronted with the threat of AIDS early in the history of the epidemic—the exercise of caution was a reflection of wisdom.[20] To others it represented an act of extraordinary timidity in the face of a lethal threat.

SHAPING POLICY IN THE FACE OF CONFLICT: 1985–1986

No controversy more sharply underscored the dilemma of how best to shape the public health policy response to AIDS in the early days of the epidemic than that which centered on gay bath houses. It was inevitable that such a controversy would emerge, since the bath houses were at once the expression of an exuberant gay sexuality, freed from the threat of state intrusion, and commercial settings within which gay men engaged in precisely those forms of anonymous sexual behavior linked to the spread of AIDS. Would the con-stitutional doctrines of privacy that had emerged in the late 1960s and 1970s protect such settings from public scrutiny, or would the demands of public health be so interpreted as to provide a warrant for their closure?

These issues first took the form of a bitter public controversy in San Fran-cisco in mid-1983.[21] For almost fifteen months public health officials, gay leaders, and civil liberties advocates were locked in conflict that riveted the attention of the nation. Only after he had obtained the support of some gay leaders did Mervyn Silverman, the city's director of public health, move to shut the baths as a public health menace. When brought before the courts, that decision was ultimately amended so that the baths could remain open but under standards that would limit the extent to which sexual behavior could occur.

This was the backdrop against which a similar battle was fought in New York City. Commissioner David Sencer had made his opposition to closure clear from the outset. "I can see no reason why we would close the bath houses. I don't think that changing the habitat is necessarily going to change the behavior. . . . To try to legislate changes in lifestyle has never been effective. Public education through the route of organized groups who are at risk is the most important thing."[22] His San Francisco counterpart, who had also initially opposed closure, ultimately moved against the baths, but Sencer never changed his mind.

Despite the opposition of the city Health Department and the virtually unanimous opposition of the leadership of New York's gay community, as well as that of the New York Civil Liberties Union, pressure for closure continued to mount. Most critically, conservative political voices demanding the bath houses be shut began to emerge. In the fall of 1985 the Republican candidate for mayor as well as the candidate of the Right-to-Life Party gave voice to such a policy.[23] It was the political origins of these demands, linked as they were to a broader opposition to the protection of gay rights, that amplified the anxiety of gay organizations about the ultimate significance of the case for closure. Ultimately, however, the liberal Democratic governor of New York State, Mario Cuomo, also called for closure.[24] Finally, in October 1985, the health commissioner of New York State announced his decision that the public health required the bath houses to be shut.[25] And so, despite the last-minute opposition of David Sencer, New York City was compelled to close institutions that permitted behaviors that everyone acknowledged were linked to the spread of the epidemic, but whose protection had taken on the symbolic significance of protecting civil liberties in the time of AIDS.

As he had displayed great caution—his opponents would term it a kind of paralysis—on the bath house issue, David Sencer also sought to prevent the embrace of other measures that might abrogate the rights of those at risk for AIDS and alienate their most vocal advocates. In mid-1985 a serological test was finally available to detect the presence of antibody to the AIDS virus.[26] First developed to screen the blood supply in order to prevent the further spread of infection to those dependent upon transfusions or antihemophelia clotting agents, it was clear virtually from the outset that such a test would also play a role in seeking to prevent the sexual transmission of HIV. Although there was some early uncertainty about the significance of a positive test finding, and considerable controversy about the adequacy of the test, these doubts were quickly resolved. When it became clear that the test was as accurate as most diagnostic tests and that a positive finding represented the presence of active HIV infection, public health officials across the country increasingly began to urge those at risk to be tested as an adjunct to counseling about behavioral change.[27] Most important, the CDC began to call for widespread voluntary confidential testing.[28] For those who feared that confidentiality would be insufficiently protected, the CDC undertook the funding of a nation-wide network of anonymous testing sites.

To gay leaders in New York as well as across the country, the test represented a great threat. Vigorous encouragement of testing would ineluctably lead to mandatory testing.[29] Those who were infected would be subject to stigmatization and deprived of the rights to work, go to school, and to obtain insurance. Some even feared that the infected would be subject to quarantines. These fears merged the historical suspicions of the gay community in a nation where half the states still criminalized homosexual behavior and the experience of AIDS-related discrimination.

In the fall of 1985, Republican Diane McGrath, who had called for the closure of the bath houses during her electoral challenge to Mayor Edward Koch, also called for mandatory testing of all teachers, food handlers, health care workers, bakers, beauticians, and prostitutes and the banning of those found to be infected from their trades.[30] Two local school boards in the borough of Queens had launched a boycott demanding that no child with AIDS be permitted to enter the classroom.[31] Hospitalized patients reported that orderlies as well as professionals were refusing to provide them with appropriate care.[32] Despite epidemiologically rooted reassurances from public health officials, public anxiety, especially in the first years of the epidemic, continued to fuel acts of discrimination that would repeatedly be denounced by health officials as unscientific, irrational, and counterproductive.

The pattern of discrimination provided the backdrop to what was to emerge as a rallying cry by gay organizations, "Don't take the test."[33] Although some gay physicians broke ranks and urged their patients who would not change behavior simply on the basis of counseling and education to be tested, for the most part gay organizations continued to express great suspicion of the HIV antibody test until the late 1980s, when the prospects for early therapeutic intervention altered the political calculus.

Sensitive to the fears of the gay community and reflecting resistance to the adoption of policies that might heighten public anxiety about the AIDS epidemic, the New York City Health Department adopted a posture unique in the nation. It alone refused to establish testing sites where individuals could seek anonymous screening. Counselors employed by the city to respond to phone calls from those anxious about AIDS tended to discourage those interested in testing from seeking such services from physicians. When, at the end of 1986, the Centers for Disease Control urged women at risk for HIV infection to be tested as a way of identifying those who could transmit AIDS to their offspring, the Health Department's Bureau of Maternity Services and Family Planning sought to issue guidelines that would have discouraged testing.[34] Mirroring the perspective of the Health Department, the Health and Hospitals Corporation, which managed the city's municipal hospitals (serving the poor and medically uninsured), sought to discourage clinicians from even offering HIV tests to patients who were free of AIDS symptoms.

It was only with regard to HIV infection among New York City's intravenous drug users that David Sencer sought to press for bold and innovative measures. Unlike those public health measures which he resisted because of concern over alienating the gay community and "pushing the epidemic underground," these were designed to lift the burden of criminalization that shaped the lives of drug users.

From the earliest days of the epidemic it was clear that those who injected drugs were at increased risk for AIDS because the needles they often shared were frequently contaminated. As early as 1984, drug sellers had begun to hawk sterile needles and syringes, or counterfeits of such equipment, at a premium, thus reflecting an awareness among users about the dangers associated with drug injection. "Get the good needles, don't get the bad AIDS."[35] Like others, Sencer began to consider the necessity of adopting policies that would permit those driven to use drugs to do so in a way that did not necessarily involve a risk of HIV transmission.

In the summer of 1985 Sencer wrote to New York's mayor urging that the laws restricting access to sterile injection equipment be radically changed.[36] "By forcing addicts to use others' needles and syringes we are condemning large numbers of addicts to death from AIDS. A live addict may be amenable to treatment of his drug abuse. But an addict infected with [the AIDS virus] continues the spread of AIDS, not only to other addicts but to their sex partners and, tragically, to children born of such parents." Although cautiously supported by the *New York Times* and the mayor, the proposal provoked an outraged response from law enforcement officials, who viewed it as a capitulation to drug abuse, a threat to the effort to contain such behavior.[37] Ultimately, the mayor yielded to such opposition. "How can I support something that the police and law enforcement leaders are totally against?"[38]

NEW LEADERSHIP, HEIGHTENED CONFLICT, AND THE POLITICS OF EPIDEMIC CONTROL: 1986–1990

The response of the city's health department to AIDS underwent a fundamental change in mid-1986 when Stephen Joseph was appointed commissioner. Joseph was by temperament more drawn to the public fray than Sencer. Thus, he sought to use his office to mobilize public concern about AIDS. Assuming office at a time when increased federal and state funds enhanced the city's capacity to confront AIDS, Joseph presided over a rapid increase in his department's budget: from $143 million in 1985 to $241 million in 1989. The funds devoted to AIDS increased from less than 1 percent of that budget to more than 7 percent; the number of staff devoted to AIDS work from 17 to over

350.[39] During Joseph's tenure the department undertook an aggressive campaign to urge individuals to seek testing for HIV infection and launched a number of blunt public information campaigns directed at heterosexuals, drug users, and gay and bisexual men.

Committed to using his office as a "bully pulpit," Joseph was nevertheless hampered by the limited functions of his department. Whatever his vision of the mission of public health in the face of the AIDS epidemic, the unique division of public health functions among the city's bureaucratic structures frustrated his efforts. In an epidemic that was increasingly rooted in drug abuse, he was without the resources or authority to expand drug abuse treatment, which since the mid-1970s had been a state prerogative. Confronted with an ever growing crisis in the provision of care to the city's poor who were afflicted with AIDS, he had virtually no capacity to expand clinical services, a responsibility that rested largely with the Health and Hospitals Corporation and ultimately with the state's Health Department. In a city where many with AIDS were dependent upon the welfare system, he had no capacity to expand the services that were the responsibility of the Human Resources Administration. In short, what was for the Department of Health the preeminent challenge was for others one of a number of social crises requiring management.

From the perspective of gay activists and others for whom AIDS was the issue confronting the city, the result was an abysmal failure.[40] The mayor was often accused of refusing to assert his leadership. So was the governor. Finally, AIDS activists recognized that it was the federal government that was responsible for much of the local failure, since it was the administration of Ronald Reagan that had presided over the epidemic's first years by resisting the introduction of adequate funding of research into treatment, support for preventive activities, and needed clinical and social services. The volunteerism that had flourished in the face of AIDS was clearly inadequate to the task of facing the city's epidemic burden. The work of the Gay Men's Health Crisis, which by the late 1980s had entailed the efforts of more than 8,000 volunteers, and other community-based groups, often created and funded by New York State to serve the city's black and Hispanic communities, were inadequate to the tasks imposed by the needs of those who were ill with HIV-related diseases.[41]

This was the context within which an explosion of rage greeted Commissioner Joseph's mid-1988 announcement that earlier estimates of the number of infected New Yorkers had been vastly overstated. Rather than 400,000 infected individuals, he asserted, the figure was closer to 200,000.[42] To those who believed that the recalculations were politically motivated there was but one explanation: in the absence of adequate services, simply declare a need for fewer services by reducing the number of infected persons. The new estimates were based on careful epdemiological modeling. But despite the belief by local and federal officials that the new statistical projections represented a more accurate picture of the extent of HIV infection in the city, the atmosphere of profound distrust that characterized the public debate of AIDS made reasoned discussion all but impossible.[43]

Most striking was the response of ACT-UP, the AIDS Coalition to Unleash Power. Disaffected by the more conventional styles of protest of mainline gay political and AIDS service organizations, ACT-UP, which adopted the pink triangle as its symbol, "Silence = Death" as its motto, relied upon the forms of direct action reminiscent of the 1960s. Joseph became the target of ACT-UP's wrath. His office was occupied by protesters, his speeches were greeted with cries of derision. Across the city, posters appeared emblazoned with a bloody hand. Because of his failures, Joseph was portrayed as being responsible for the deaths of thousands.

If the gay community was alienated from Joseph because of his "epidemiological politics," the city's minority community was outraged by his insistence that David Sencer's proposal for needle exchange be subjected to an experimental trial. Resisted for more than a year by the state's health officials, the proposal for such an experiment ultimately received the necessary approval on the condition that it be small and serve only as a bridge to treatment for addicts awaiting admission to conventional therapeutic programs.[44] Scheduled to begin in the fall of 1988, the needle plan, in which addicts would be required to exchange used drug injection equipment for sterile paraphernalia, produced a bitter reaction from the city's black and Hispanic leadership. Benjamin Ward, the black police commissioner denounced it as the equivalent of the infamous Tuskegee syphilis experiment.[45] In a letter published in the *Amsterdam News*, New York's leading black newspaper, and signed by Harlem's congressional representative, Charles Rangel, Queens representative Floyd Flake, Sterling Johnson (the special assistant district attorney for drug prosecutions), Wyatt Walker (the pastor of Harlem's Covenant Baptist Church), and Wilbert Tatum (publisher of the *Amsterdam News*), the plan was denounced as "a very serious mistake" that would represent the first step toward legalizing drugs. The Black and Hispanic Caucus of the City Council also denounced the proposal, declaring it "beyond all human reason and common sense." One black councilman termed the proposal genocidal and declared, "When the first needle is given out by Dr. Joseph, he ought to be indicted and arrested for murder and drug distribution."[46] Finally, community groups opposed the planned use of neighborhood health clinics as distribution points since centers would inevitably be too close to public schools.

Despite the expressions of distrust and vilification, the Commissioner, backed by the mayor, opened the first clinic in November 1988. Because of the community-based opposition, all needle exchange was centralized at the

Health Department's offices in the shadow of the Criminal Court Building. And so began a much-hobbled initiative that resembled David Sencer's initial proposal in only the remotest way.

The bitterness about the course of AIDS prevention policy during Stephen Joseph's tenure found its final expression in the summer of 1989. Convinced that the strategy of AIDS prevention in the epidemic's first years had failed to call effectively upon the tradition of public health epidemic control, and motivated by the prospects opened up by the rapid development of therapeutics in 1989, which suggested that early clinical intervention could slow the development of lethal disease in those infected with HIV, Stephen Joseph sought to chart a new direction. Using the venue of the Fifth International AIDS Conference in Montreal, he declared that it was time to begin "a shift toward a disease control approach to HIV infection along the lines of classic tuberculosis practice."[47] A central feature of such an approach would be the "reporting of seropositives" to assure effective clinical follow-up and the initiation of "more aggressive contact tracing."

To gay leaders and advocates of civil liberties, Joseph's embrace of traditional public health practice, involving a more aggressive reliance on screening, the reporting of the names of infected persons to the Department of Health, contact tracing, and the selective use of the power to quarantine when infected persons continued to behave in ways that placed sexual or needle-sharing partners at risk, represented a profound assault on what they had come to believe was the appropriate strategy for confronting the AIDS epidemic—a strategy that recognized the centrality of the protection of the right of privacy. Marshaling evidence from studies across the nation that suggested that compulsory reporting of HIV infection would discourage individuals from coming forward for testing, they argued that the proposed new course would have the unintended consequence of driving individuals away from testing, precisely at a moment when clinical advances suggested that they seek testing. To groups such as GMHC, which had just undertaken a radical rethinking of their antagonism to testing, the commissioner's call seemed a special insult.

Joseph's proposal—in truth a reflection of the reconsideration of mandatory reporting by many public health officials—opened a debate that was only temporarily settled by the defeat of New York Mayor Edward Koch in his bid for reelection in the fall of 1989. When newly elected Mayor David Dinkins, who as the city's first black mayor had relied upon the support of New York's gay voters, announced the appointment of Woodrow Myers, Indiana's black commissioner of health, as Joseph's replacement, the issue resurfaced. Myers had supported named reporting in Indiana.[48] Now the controversy took on distinctly racial overtones. White gay leaders and their liberal political allies opposed Myers's appointment when his past policies became known. To black leaders this opposition represented an insult to the black mayor and an assault on his right to shape a new administration. The controversy, which left many embittered and some saddened, was brought to a close only when Dinkins announced that, despite the opposition of some gay leaders and especially that of ACT-UP, Myers would be the City's health commissioner, although there would be no reporting of the names of those with HIV infection.[49]

The truce was once again shattered when Commissioner Myers, fulfilling a promise made by Dinkins during his campaign, ended the city's small needle exchange program.[50] Liberals and gay leaders, who had enthusiastically endorsed this aspect of Stephen Joseph's AIDS policy, were thus presented with a profound disappointment at the hands of the mayoral candidate they had supported. Disappointment turned to dismay when in the late spring of 1990 Commissioner Myers sought to cancel a small municipal contract with ADAPT, a community-based organization committed to educating drug users about AIDS prevention, because part of its effort involved the distribution of bleach for the sterilization of injection equipment.[51] An approach to working with drug users that had rarely provoked opposition anyplace in the United States except from the most socially conservative, bleach education and distribution had attained an important symbolic status for those who sought to fashion policies designed to inhibit the spread of HIV infection.

In challenging such programs, Myers had made it clear that he had priorities beyond those of preventing HIV transmission—some began to wonder whether AIDS would be a priority of his at all. "There's a higher goal than the reduction of transmission of HIV and that goal is the elimination of the use of illegal narcotics by injection, period. . . . I just happen to believe very strongly that people who are using drugs ought to stop using drugs." As a consequence, he opposed efforts to "teach them how to use drugs safely."[52] Myers's position reflected the views of the city's black and Hispanic leadership. His decision reflected the changing balance of power in local AIDS politics. Myers's action was supported by the Black Leadership Commission on AIDS, which saw the distribution of bleach as a "Trojan horse for the African American Community" and as failing to address the root causes of drug use and the scarcity of drug rehabilitation programs.[53] Myers's effort to cancel the city's contract with ADAPT provoked a sharp reaction from white AIDS activists in ACT-UP as well as from liberal political leaders, some of whom referred to it as "genocidal."[54] What this controversy underscored was the deepening fissure between the gay and white liberal constituencies that had helped to shape the broad outlines of AIDS policies in the epidemic's first decade and the ascendant leadership of the black community that sought to define a strategy appropriate to an epidemic that was increasingly taking on the dimensions of a dire problem for the city's impoverished black and Hispanic communities.

The conflict between the city's gay community and the health department abated with the sudden resignation of Myers, who had proved to be a poor manager. His replacement, Margaret Hamburg, found a department in disarray, many of its most talented officers had been forced to resign or had left their positions in despair. Most important, Hamburg was not committed to the ideological posture that had characterized her predecessor. With evidence mounting on the potential efficacy of needle exchange programs—most strikingly from New Haven, which had undertaken a trial effort under the leadership of a black mayor—she was instrumental in moving Mayor David Dinkins to a more open position on the matter.

A confluence of factors, including a reversal of the position of the Black Leadership Commission; the incapacitation of the state's health commissioner, who had been unsympathetic to needle exchange; a major funding initiative for community-based needle exchange programs by the American Foundation for AIDS Research (AmFAR); and the acquittal on grounds of "necessity" of several ACT-UP members who had been arrested for illegal distribution of sterile injection equipment, cleared the way for the beginning of legal needle exchange efforts in New York City. In 1992, three such programs were functioning at a variety of locales in the city. Funded by the State Health Department and AmFAR, these efforts failed to provoke the outrage that had greeted the efforts of Stephen Joseph four years earlier. Remarkably, the opposition of the black community had all but vanished.

CARING FOR THE SICK: THE PRICE OF NEGLECT

The initial response of the city's black and Hispanic leadership to proposals for needle exchange must be viewed in the context of rising anger and despair over the city's failure to provide an adequate rehabilitative response to the problem of heroin, cocaine, and crack abuse. There were in New York City something more than thirty thousand treatment positions for the more than two hundred thousand drug injectors and many thousands more who used crack and other drugs. This failure was in turn a reflection of the unwillingness of both the state and federal governments to provide the necessary funding for such services. But such inadequacy was but a small part of a much broader problem: the inadequacy of funds to provide for the medical services needed to meet the clinical needs of the rising number of patients with AIDS-related disorders. As the importance of early prophylactic treatment with AZT (for slowing the progression of viral infection) and pentamidine (for inhibiting the occurrence of pneumocystis pneumonia) became clear in mid-1989, the crisis in health care became all the more obvious. It was not only those with frank disease who would now need care, but the much larger group of individuals with asymptomatic HIV infection.

As early as the spring of 1988, the dimensions of the impending crisis were already. clear. Investigators writing in the *Bulletin of the New York Academy of Medicine* thus noted that "to ignore the possibilities inherent in the empirical evidence available is to create a social calamity even greater than the one already perceived. . . . The AIDS epidemic threatens not only individual lives but the city's health care, education and research environment as well. The time is short, the need is great and is likely to grow rapidly."[55] Within a year three separate reports by public- or voluntary-sector groups detailed how far New York was from being able to meet the demands of the epidemic.[56] All agreed that community-based organizations, typically within the gay community, had provided an extraordinary range of services to those with HIV infection and AIDS but could not meet the needs that public bodies and large private-sector agencies were responsible for meeting. Volunteerism was no substitute for the institutional response that was demanded. Three to five hundred new acute-care hospital beds would be needed each year for five years in order to meet the requirements of those who would become ill. In addition, hundreds of nursing home beds and special housing units would be needed for those requiring less-intensive medical care. The capital costs alone for meeting these demands would be over $700 million. And if only half of those who could benefit from ambulatory care for HIV infection were to seek it, the city's already overburdened clinic system would have to absorb an additional eight hundred thousand visits a year. Commenting on the care and attention to detail revealed in each of the report projections, Kenneth Raske, president of the Greater New York Hospital Association, said, "This is the biggest amount of planning for an epidemic with the least amount of action to go along with it."[57]

When the state of New York, upon which the city was so financially dependent for health care services, announced its five-year plan for AIDS in early 1989, Governor Mario Cuomo acknowledged that he was not able to provide the funds to meet the state's goals "realistically." Liberal political leaders denounced the governor's fiscal restraint. Richard Gottfried, chair of the state assembly's health committee, termed the governor's proposed budget "a blueprint for disaster."[58] ACT-UP turned to the streets. Approximately three thousand demonstrators chanting "ACT-UP/Fight Back/Fight AIDS" appeared at City Hall. Two hundred were arrested.[59]

The looming crisis in health care in New York as well as in other cities across the United States set the stage for congressional action in 1990 that could scarcely have been imagined a short time earlier. It was the fruit of dogged efforts on the part of AIDS activists, their allies, and some political leaders from the cities and states that had borne the disproportionate share of AIDS cases. In the winter of 1990, Senator Edward Kennedy, the exemplar of Democratic party liberalism, and Senator Orrin Hatch, a Republican whose stance on abortion often cast him in the role of a conservative, jointly sponsored legislation—Comprehensive AIDS Resource Emergency Act of 1990—that would provide a major infusion of federal assistance to those localities most severely burdened by AIDS. "The Human Immunodeficiency

Virus constitutes a crisis as devastating as an earthquake, flood or drought. Indeed, the death toll of the unfolding AIDS tragedy is already a hundredfold greater han any natural disaster to strike our nation in this century."[60]

As remarkable as the joint sponsorship of this legislation, which promised to provide $2.9 billion over five years in a complex political formula to the cities and states most severely struck by AIDS, was the overwhelming support the legislation received in the Senate, where the vote in favor was 95-4. When similar legislation, with even greater resource commitments, was voted on by the House of Representatives, the vote was 408-14.[61]

But the hopes of early summer 1990 were dashed by the fall as the Congress, confronted with a severe budgetary crisis, slashed funds for what was now called the Ryan White Act.

The limits of this federal initiative will inevitably have a profound impact on the capacity of New York City to manage the ever-growing burden posed by the AIDS epidemic. As the city and state began to confront new fiscal crises in the latter part of 1990, it was clear that capacity would be subject to even greater strain. In the spring of 1990 there were already signs of what the future might bring. Several clinics created to treat people with HIV infection had waiting lists of up to three months. Two clinics had closed their waiting lists, and only 13,000 of the estimated 40,000 to 140,000 who could benefit from AZT, the only licensed antiviral agent, were receiving it.[62]

For close observers of the chronic but escalating crisis in health care in New York City, it was not too soon to start thinking of worst-case scenarios.[63] They began to argue publicly that the impact of AIDS would affect the ability of the city's medical and social service infrastructure to provide care not only to those with HIV infection but to others as well. As a consequence, middle-class patients together with their physicians might increasingly flee the city in search of medical care in the suburbs. If they remained and were able to protect their own interests by insulating themselves from the critical shortage of hospital beds, those institutions forced to bear the burden of caring for the poor would be compelled to restrict even further access to in-patient care for "elective" procedures. While middle-class patients with HIV infection would continue to receive increasingly effective outpatient care from their overworked physicians, the poor would face growing delays and waiting lists as they sought the benefits of early therapeutic intervention. Many, discouraged, would simply not seek care at all.

Shortages would impose the need for rationing, and in the political economy of a city like New York, competition among the desperate would ensue. In what Bruce Vladeck, then president of the United Hospital Fund, and now the assistant secretary of the federal Health Care Finance Agency, termed the "calculus of misery," it would become increasingly necessary to choose between AIDS cases and the frail elderly for admission to nursing homes; between single adults with AIDS and homeless families with young children for access to newly renovated apartments; between homeless persons dying of AIDS and children for access to transitional shelter; between HIV-infected pregnant women and women not yet infected for admission to drug abuse treatment programs.

New York, the epicenter of the American epidemic, yet dependent upon resources from the state and federal governments, would thus witness not only a grave medical challenge but increasingly aggravated social conditions as it prepared to face the second decade of AIDS.

ENVOI: THE RETURN OF TUBERCULOSIS

In 1992 the attention of public health officials as well as the media was seized by a new HIV-related challenge, the resurgence of tuberculosis, a disease that had long been thought tightly under control. Socially rooted in the rise of homelessness, untreated drug addiction, and a swelling prison population, the rise in new cases of tuberculosis was centrally linked as well to the AIDS epidemic. Those with HIV infection are, because of compromised immune systems, at vastly greater risk of developing TB once infected with *micobacterium* tuberculosis than those who are not dually infected. As a consequence, the epidemics were epidemiologically joined.

But it was the singular unpreparedness—despite the fact that TB cases had been rising since the early 1980s—on the part of the public health system that made the rising incidence of TB so perilous. Underfunded and understaffed, the city's TB control apparatus was utterly incapable of monitoring the treatment of those with disease. As a result, drug-resistant strains became ever more common. By April 1991, 20 percent of those diagnosed with tuberculosis in New York were resistant to treatment by Rifampin and Isoniazid, the two antibiotics most relied upon for TB treatment. While most drug resistant cases occurred in individuals who had failed to complete an initial course of therapy, there were indications that resistant organisms were being transmitted to those who had never had tuberculosis. The overall case fatality rate for drug-resistant tuberculosis was 40–60 percent—precisely the case fatality of untreated drug-susceptible TB. In those cases where resistant strains were transmitted to individuals with HIV infection, the outcome was almost universally fatal.

Thus poverty, the AIDS epidemic, and the fiscal crisis in New York that so limited the responsiveness of the public health system threatened, in 1992, to turn a formerly treatable disease into a virulent new threat to all New Yorkers, but most especially to those infected with HIV.

Notes

1. Centers for Disease Control (hereafter CDC), "Pneumocystis Pneumonia—Los Angeles," *Morbidity Mortality Weekly Report* (hereafter *MMWR*) (June 5, 1981): 250–252.

2. CDC, "Kaposi's Sarcoma and Pneumocystis Pneumonia among Homosexual Men—New York City and California," *MMWR* (July 3, 1981): 305–308.

3. Pauline Thomas et al., "HIV Infection in Heterosexual Female Intravenous Drug Users in New York City," *New England Journal of Medicine* (August 11, 1988): 374.

4. Don Des Jarlais et al., "HIV-I Infection among Intravenous Drug Users in Manhattan, New York City, from 1977–1987," *Journal of the American Medical Association* (February 17, 1989): 1009.

5. "Report of the Expert Panel of HIV Seroprevalence Estimates and AIDS Case Projection Methodologies" (February 1989, mimeographed).

6. New York City Department of Health, Office of AIDS Surveillance, "AIDS Surveillance Update Second Quarter 1992" (July 31, 1992, mimeographed).

7. Ernest Drucker and Sten Vermund, "Estimating Population Prevalence of HIV Infection in Urban Areas with High Rates of Drug Use, A Model of the Bronx in 1988," *American Journal of Epidemiology* 130, no. 1 (1989): 133–142.

8. New York State Department of Health, "HIV Seroprevalence Study" (July 1, 1988, mimeographed).

9. New York City Department of Health, "AIDS Surveillance Update" (September 26, 1990).

10. *New York Native*, March 29–April 11, 1982, 15.

11. *New York Native*, June 21–July 4, 1982, 11.

12. See, for example, Jonathan Lieberson, "Anatomy of an Epidemic," *New York Review of Books* (August 18, 1983): 19.

13. *New York Native*, January 12–30, 1983, 5.

14. *New York Native*, March 14–27, 1983, 1.

15. Peter Arno and Robert Hughes, "Local Policy Responses to the AIDS Epidemic: New York and San Francisco," *New York State Journal of Medicine* (May 1987): 264–272.

16. Harlon Dalton, "AIDS in Blackface," *Daedalus* (Summer 1989): part I.

17. Sam Friedman et al., "The AIDS Epidemic among Blacks and Hispanics," *Milbank Quarterly* 65, suppl. 2 (1987): 490.

18. Arno and Hughes, "Local Policy Responses," 268.

19. Richard Neustadt and Harvey Fineberg, *The Epidemic That Never Was* (New York: Vintage Books, 1983).

20. Ronald Bayer, *Private Acts, Social Consequences: AIDS and the Politics of Public Health* (New Brunswick, N.J.: Rutgers University Press, 1991).

21. Ibid., 31–53.

22. Lieberson, "Anatomy of an Epidemic," 21.

23. *New York Times*, October 30, 1985; *New York Times*, October 5, 1985.

24. *New York Times*, October 30, 1985.

25. *New York Times*, October 25, 1985.

26. CDC, "Provisional Public Health Service Inter-Agency Recommendations for

Screening Donated Blood and Plasma for Antibody to the Virus Causing Acquired Immunodeficiency Syndrome," *MMWR* (January 11, 1985): 1–5.

27. Association of State and Territorial Health Officials (ASTHO), *ASTHO Guide to Public Health Practice: HTLV III Antibody Testing and Community Approaches* (Washington, D.C.: Public Health Foundation, 1985).

28. CDC, "Additional Recommendations to Reduce Sexual and Drug Abuse-Related Transmission of Human T-Lymphotropic Virus Type III/Lymphadenopathy-Associated Virus," *MMWR* (March 14, 1986): 152–155.

29. American Association of Physicians for Human Rights, *Newsletter* (November 1985).

30. *New York Times*, October 2, 1985.

31. David Kirp, *Learning by Heart* (New Brunswick, N.J.: Rutgers University Press, 1990).

32. Ronald Bayer, "AIDS and the Duty to Treat: Risk, Responsibility and Health Care Workers," *Bulletin of the New York Academy of Medicine* (July–August 1988): 498–505.

33. *New York Native*, October 8–21, 1984, 1.

34. CDC, "Recommendations for Assisting in the Prevention of Perinatal Transmission of Human T-Lymphotropic Virus III/Lymphadenopathy-Associated Virus and Acquired Immunodeficiency Syndrome," *MMWR* (December 6, 1986): 721–726, 731–32; Committee on Perinatal Transmission of Human T-Lymphotropic Virus Type III/Lymphadenopathy-Associated Virus, New York City Department of Health, Bureau of Maternity Services and Family Planning, Report (Mimeographed, n.d).

35. Don Des Jarlais et al., "Epidemiology and Risk Reduction for AIDS among Intravenous Drug Users," *Annals of Internal Medicine* (November 1985): 758.

36. David Sencer memorandum to Edward Koch, August 13, 1985.

37. *New York Times,* May 30, 1985.

38. *New York Times,* May 30, 1986.

39. Ellen Rautenberg, assistant commissioner of health for AIDS program services, January 8, 1990, personal communication.

40. Charles Perrow, *The AIDS Disaster: The Failure of Organization in New York and the Nation* (New Haven, Conn.: Yale University Press, 1990).

41. Suzanne Oullette Kobasa, "AIDS and Volunteer Associations: Perspective on Social and Individual Changing," *Milbank Quarterly*, suppl. 2 (1990): 280–294.

42. *New York Times,* September 23, 1988, A14.

43. "Report of the Expert Panel on HIV Seroprevalence Estimates and AIDS Case Projection Methodologies" (February 1989, mimeographed).

44. Stephen C. Joseph, "A Bridge to Treatment: The Needle Exchange Pilot Program in New York City," *AIDS Education and Prevention* 1, no. 4 (1989): 340–345.

45. *New York Post*, October 31, 1988.

46. *New York Daily News,* October 28, 1988.

47. Stephen C. Joseph, "Remarks at the Fifth International Conference on AIDS" (June 5, 1989, mimeographed).

48. *American Medical News*, May 18, 1990, 3.

49. Ibid.

50. *New York Times*, April 10, 1990.

51. *New York Newsday*, May 6, 1990.

52. Ibid.

53. *New York Newsday*, June 16, 1990.

54. *New York Newsday*, June 8, 1990.

55. Michael Alderman et al., "Predicting the Future of the AIDS Epidemic and Its Consequences for the Health Care System of New York City," *Bulletin of the New York Academy of Medicine* (March 1988): 181.

56. New York City AIDS Task Force, *Report* (July 1989); Citizens Commission on AIDS, *The Crisis in AIDS Care* (March 1989); Mayor's Task Force on AIDS, *Assuring Care for New York City's AIDS Population* (March 1989).

57. *New York Times*, April 23, 1989.

58. *New York Times*, February 16, 1989.

59. *New York Times*, March 29, 1989.

60. Senator Edward Kennedy, letter, February 1990, mimeographed.

61. *New York Times*, June 14, 1990.

62. *New York Newsday*, April 14, 1990.

63. United Hospital Fund, "President's Letter" (February 1990).

III

The City
Responds

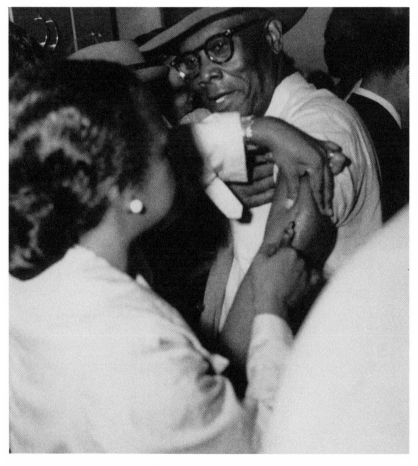

Interior of mobile Salk polio vaccination clinic operated by the New York City Department of Health, as an adult took advantage of the free Salk polio shot made available to him. New York, August 4, 1959. Collection of March of Dimes Birth Defects Foundation.

Until the formation of the Metropolitan Board of Health, New Yorkers responded to epidemics much as any culture responds to emergencies: temporary measures were instituted by hastily organized quasi-governmental bodies. During the early yellow fever and cholera outbreaks, for example, the mayor appointed temporary boards of health that organized for the duration of the epidemic quarantines, fumigation, street cleaning, and prayer meetings. When the epidemic subsided, the board disbanded.

The creation of the Metropolitan Board of Health in 1866 marked a distinct change in the administration of public health and was an implicit acknowledgment of the disintegration of the city's health during the previous decades. No longer could politicians or the city's population ignore epidemic disease or feel secure in the belief that disease would be confined to poor neighborhoods, specific communities of immigrant, or the wharves and docks of lower Manhattan. It was also an acknowledgment of the changing perception of the health crisis: By mid-century, disease was endemic in and native to the city. It was not a periodic, unwelcome, or foreign visitor.

By the late nineteenth century, New York's public health agencies were reacting to the growing prominence of the laboratory and the sophistication of bacteriology as a field. The association of specific germs with particular disease entities spurred public health officials to adopt new practices and methods in addressing epidemic disease. Especially important was the development of new techniques capable of producing large quantities of vaccines and antitoxins capable of treating such frightening childhood scourges as diphtheria. Yet the very activities that provided such promise also became part of larger political dramas then overtaking the department, local physicians, the city political machines. The department, despite its protestations to the contrary, was part of city government, and the government's political culture and concerns, ranging from jobs through infringements of civil liberties, directly affected the department's activities. The first essay in this section, by Fee and Hammonds, provides a glimpse into the politics of public health practice and the place of technical change in that process. Further, Fee and Hammonds identify the growing role of a commercial culture that gave individuals in the department room to turn scientific discoveries into personal gain. Similarly, the impact of the early struggles around the place of bacteriology and the laboratory served to broaden the scope and definition of public health practice. The department emerged as preeminent and as a model for others throughout the country.

The expanding scope of public health activities since the 1920s is detailed in Daniel M. Fox's chapter, which concludes this volume. The essay reminds us of the dangers of memory in detailing the history of public health. The view of some historians that the early twentieth century marked the zenith of public health practice ignores the shifting and complex redefinition of public health that has emerged in the years since then. Fox reminds us that we now see the field much more broadly and that activities as varied as hospital care and insurance policy are now included as part of public health's political, scientific, and academic agenda. One need only look at the annual program of the American Public Health Association or its New York affiliate, the Public Health Association of New York City (PHANYC), to understand how broad that definition is. Significantly, many of the activities of public health take place outside the political and institutional framework of the Department of Health, especially in the decades following World War II when public health officials appeared to agree that "major epidemics [had] disappeared." Voluntary associations, federal and state agencies, and various other city departments all have a role in the broader health agenda. As Bayer pointed out in "The Dependent Center" earlier in this volume, few would argue that the Health and Hospitals Corporation of the city or the welfare department are not involved in public health policy around AIDS. By the beginning of this latest major epidemic, authority and function in the field of public health had been dispersed among a large number of actors, agencies, and institutions.

ELIZABETH FEE AND EVELYNN M. HAMMONDS

Science, Politics, and the Art of Persuasion: Promoting the New Scientific Medicine in New York City

In 1901, Robert Koch, the most revered of the German bacteriologists, wrote to Hermann Biggs to congratulate the New York City Department of Health for having achieved the compulsory reporting of tuberculosis: "I wish to cite the example of the free American people who of their own free will accepted the limitation of their own liberties for the sake of public health."[1] This curious compliment came less than twenty years after the 1882 announcement of Koch's discovery of the tubercle bacillus and was heady recognition indeed for New York's practical accomplishments in applying the new science of bacteriology.

Americans, who had for so long trailed behind Europe's scientific superiority, were now beginning to be noticed for their contributions to public health.[2] Befitting America's reputation as a country of practical and pragmatic orientation, the New York bacteriological laboratory's main claim to fame was its ability to translate theoretical discoveries into successful techniques for the diagnosis, prevention, and treatment of disease. Here, bacteriology imported from Europe was used to transform public health practice. In promoting bacteriological methods, public health officials would make innovative use of the media in raising money, gaining the support (or at least acquiescence) of politicians, and rousing the interest of the general public—thus demonstrating the peculiar amalgam of science and politics that characterizes all successful innovation in public health.

New York City was not the first American city to develop a bacteriological laboratory; that credit goes to Lawrence, Massachusetts; Ann Arbor, Michigan; and Providence, Rhode Island.[3] These earlier laboratories, however, had been primarily devoted to the analysis of food and water; New York's was the first routinely used to diagnose disease. The New York bacteriological laboratory's success in applying bacteriological techniques was aided by the relative autonomy of the city's health department. Unlike those of Britain or other European countries, New York's health department was established as an independent organization, with the broadest possible powers over all matters connected with the scientific investigation, diagnosis, care, and sanitary supervision of infectious diseases.[4]

The story of the bacteriological laboratory formally begins on September 13, 1892, when, under intense pressure and fearing an impending cholera epidemic, the New York Board of Health agreed to create a new Division of Pathology, Bacteriology, and Disinfection.[5] Under the direction of the dynamic Hermann M. Biggs, this division would outlast the immediate concern with cholera and expand to deal with other infectious diseases: diphtheria, tuberculosis, typhoid fever, smallpox, and infant diarrhea. It would help shift the central focus of public health practice from concern with the cleanliness of the urban environment to the diagnosis and treatment of specific diseases. As we will see, this shift would bring public health into much closer relationship with medical practice and provoke struggles for power and authority between public health officials and private practitioners.

Before the establishment of the bacteriological laboratories in the 1890s, public health practice in New York, as in other American cities, was largely a matter of sanitary engineering.[6] When the New York State legislature originally approved the city's autonomous Board of Health on February 26, 1866, the board began a heroic effort to clean up the city and eliminate the worst sanitary abuses.[7] In 1870, the board was replaced by a Department of Health with four bureaus: the Bureau of Sanitary Inspection, the Bureau of Records and Inspection, the Bureau of Street Cleaning, and the Sanitary Permit Bureau. This organization reflected the central importance of sanitation, inspection, and street cleaning, activities intended to prevent disease by reducing the poisonous exhalations (miasmas) emitted by decomposing organic matter.[8]

AMERICAN RESPONSES TO THE NEW SCIENCE OF BACTERIOLOGY

By 1880, American physicians were divided in their responses to the new germ theory being advanced in Europe; by the mid-1880s, bacteriology had begun to establish itself as a legitimate science in a small number of American medical schools.[9] Patricia Gossel notes that Koch's announcement of the discovery of the tubercle bacillus in 1882 had an electrifying effect on the American medical community; before that date, few physicians thought the germ theory deserved much credibility.[10] Now everyone with access to a laboratory wanted to try to confirm or refute Koch's discovery. Although many Americans could now stain slides and identify bacteria under the microscope in some crude fashion, Koch's more subtle techniques were difficult to duplicate.

Those wanting to become serious bacteriologists had to travel abroad for specialized training, preferably in Germany, where renowned authorities taught students the latest concepts and techniques.[11]

Three of the young Americans who made the pilgrimage to Germany were T. Mitchell Prudden, William Henry Welch, and Hermann M. Biggs.[12] All were to play major roles in the introduction of bacteriological research to the United States.[13] Welch established laboratories at Bellevue Hospital and the Johns Hopkins Medical School, Prudden at the Columbia College of Physicians and Surgeons, and Biggs in the New York City Health Department. Welch's main role in the New York story would be as Biggs's teacher, mentor, and supporter, and as a national authority to be invoked in moments of crisis.[14]

When William Henry Welch and T. Mitchell Prudden returned to New York after studying in Germany, they initially devoted themselves to research and teaching in pathology; the two young men then turned their attention to bacteriology when they heard Koch's announcement in 1882 that he had identified the specific bacillus causing tuberculosis. In 1885, both Welch and Prudden returned to Berlin to study bacteriology in an intensive month-long course with Koch himself.[15] Back in the United States, Prudden argued that public health departments must establish laboratories to study bacteria in relation to disease.[16] Local and national health boards, he declared, should be leaders in bacteriological research, and in the testing, diagnosis, and treatment of disease—a view based on his observations of Koch's model, the Imperial Department of Health in Berlin.[17]

Prudden was appointed consulting pathologist to the New York City Health Department in 1887, and in 1889 coauthored a major report with Alfred Loomis and Hermann Biggs on tuberculosis; they argued that if the disease was transmitted by a bacillus, it should be preventable.[18] They recommended inspecting all cattle providing milk or meat to New York City, disinfecting any premises occupied by tuberculosis patients, and teaching people that the disease was spread by human contact.

Like Welch and Prudden, Hermann Biggs had been greatly stimulated by Koch's discovery. Even as an undergraduate, he had been interested in public health. His baccalaureate thesis of 1882, written when he was twenty-three, was a rather magisterial document on "Sanitary Regulations and the Duty of the State in Relation to Public Hygiene." In it he argued that government support for public health was key to maintaining the physical, moral, and intellectual condition of the community.[19] Biggs studied under Welch at Bellevue Hospital Medical College, spent several months in German laboratories, and then became first assistant at the newly established Carnegie Laboratory in New York.[20] At the Carnegie Laboratory, he confirmed Koch's identification of the comma bacillus as diagnostic of "Asiatic" cholera and published papers on tuberculosis and typhoid fever. In 1885, Andrew Carnegie sent him to Paris, with four children who had been bitten by a rabid dog, to study Pasteur's new method for the treatment of rabies.[21]

Biggs also worked as a consultant to the New York City Health Department in testing the efficacy of sulphur dioxide as a disinfectant for the clothes and belongings of immigrants. Biggs was soon to have a chance to try his skills at bacteriological diagnosis in 1887, when a young boy from a quarantined ship died of suspected Asiatic cholera. It was difficult to distinguish the fatal and epidemic Asiatic cholera symptomatically from the milder, nonepidemic form of sporadic cholera. In his laboratory, however, Biggs could identify the characteristic comma bacillus and thus confirm that the boy had died of the more severe form of the disease. In his report of the incident, Biggs claimed that the bacteriological examination had kept epidemic cholera out of New York City.[22] As an effective publicist, Biggs was already arguing that the city should establish and fund a bacteriological laboratory to protect the public's health.

In 1887, Biggs and Prudden were consulting pathologists to the Health Department; they also served on an advisory committee to the New York Academy of Medicine to study the establishment of a quarantine post on Hoffman Island. Their interest in applying bacteriology to public health was already clear; the question was whether and how they could parlay an occasional consulting position, prompted by the immediate threat of impending epidemics, into regular and permanent appointments that would allow them to develop a real scientific and political base in the city.

POLITICAL SCANDAL AND THE THREAT OF CHOLERA

The catalyst for change was the peculiar conjuncture of a cholera epidemic threatening New York in 1892 and a political scandal affecting the Health Department. First came the political problems. In the summer of 1892, the press had been paying close attention to the machinations of Tammany Hall and specifically to accusations that recent personnel changes in the Health Department were the result of political manipulation. On June 25, 1892, a group of prominent physicians belonging to the Medical Advisory Board of the Board of Health resigned. In a fairly unusual move, two of the members of the advisory board, Abraham Jacobi and T. Mitchell Prudden, publicly announced that they were resigning because the Health Department had fallen into the hands of a political machine, Tammany Hall.[23]

Charles Wilson, the president of the Board of Health, denied that he had been subject to outside pressure and claimed to have replaced Sanitary Superintendent Ewing and demoted the registrar of records "for the good of the department."[24] The city physicians were unconvinced. On June 29, the prominent physician and sanitary reformer Dr. Stephen Smith also resigned his consulting position, while noting that the original agreement with the Medical

Advisory Board had been that politics would be kept out of public health work: "Politics was to be absolutely avoided in order that the best professional service could be fearlessly rendered to the city. . . . Eventually a change was made by which a layman became eligible to the presidency of the Board. This naturally led to a politician being placed in that office and to a department being turned into a part of the patronage dispensing machine apparently inseparable from political work."[25] By July 6, 1892, the remaining members of the Medical Advisory Board had resigned.

Physicians in New York had long opposed the appointment of lay members to the Board of Health, especially to the presidency. In their view, professional prerogatives and defense of the public good both demanded that the medical profession exercise authority over public health matters. They did not want the profession divided by partisan politics; physicians knew that it was in their collective interest to avoid being tainted by association with political machines. Health Commissioner Joseph D. Bryant worked long and hard to improve relations between the Health Department and the medical profession and had set up the Medical Advisory Board precisely to gain more support for public health efforts from physicians.[26]

Bryant's hard work seemed to have gone for naught in the wake of the scandal of 1892. The *New York Tribune* declared that "Tammany's relentless pursuit of spoils has seldom been more strikingly and repulsively illustrated than in the recent manipulation of the Health Board," while the *New York Times* warned of dire long-term consequences: "The Board of Health cannot be used as a political machine in the service of Tammany Hall, or managed under the sway of the dictation of politicians, without driving from its assistance all physicians of high standing in the community."[27] Reform political groups, interested in overthrowing the power of Tammany to control municipal government, used the resignations of the Medical Advisory Board in their public campaign. The City Reform Club sent out between twenty-five thousand and thirty thousand copies of a leaflet entitled "Politics in the Health Department," deploring the recent firings and explaining the resignations of the medical board. It also reprinted the text of an editorial from the *New York Medical Journal* attacking Charles Wilson: "Any Board of Health—in this city or any other—that has for its head a mere politician is like a pyramid built upon its apex instead of its base."[28]

By the middle of August 1892, all members of the Consulting Medical Board, except for Dr. George Shrady, had resigned, and T. Mitchell Prudden had resigned as consulting pathologist.[29] Asked by the City Reform Club about his reasons for resigning, Prudden explained, "A general and growing distrust of the methods of the health board under its present head and his wardens in those departments which I had occasion to know most about . . . have led me for some time to wish to free myself from all further association with it."[30] Another physician wrote in an anonymous letter to the editor of the *New York*

Medical Journal, "It has been an open secret for years that appointment as surgeons to the police force (notwithstanding the examination), to the various medical positions in the Board of Health and to the non-remunerative positions as members of the visiting staff of the various municipal hospitals were matters of political influence."[31]

Two notable persons who did not resign their positions in the summer of 1892 were the health commissioner, Joseph Bryant, and the consulting pathologist, Hermann Biggs. Bryant held a secure position in the Health Department and had survived other attacks from Tammany. We can only speculate about the reasons Biggs stayed in his post. Perhaps it was loyalty to Bryant, his teacher and mentor. Perhaps his attention was focused on the increasingly numerous reports of cholera outbreaks in Europe. By August 1892, Asiatic cholera had reached Hamburg, a major point of departure for immigrants to the United States, and had already caused thousands of deaths in a devastating epidemic. It seemed inevitable that the disease would reach New York. Bryant and Biggs may have realized they could benefit by staying and gaining leverage with Wilson and the Board of Aldermen. Wilson would want to defuse the negative publicity the department had received all summer and might now be willing to back Bryant and Biggs's previously unsuccessful proposal to establish a special division of bacteriology and disinfection. The news of cholera from Europe added growing urgency to the situation.

On August 30, the steamship *Moravia* arrived from Hamburg with news that twenty-two passengers had already been buried at sea after succumbing to severe intestinal attacks.[32] The surviving passengers were transferred to a quarantine station, where they and their luggage were scrubbed, fumigated, and disinfected. New York City at first reacted to the impending threat of cholera in traditional ways, by thoroughly cleaning its streets and conducting increased health inspections of tenements, food, and water supplies.

City leaders needed to assure the public that everything possible was being done to protect the city from cholera. On August 31, Hermann Biggs was called in to conduct bacteriological examinations to determine the cause of the deaths on the *Moravia.* That same day, President Charles Wilson showed reporters around the chemical laboratory at 42 Bleeker Street, which supposedly had been improved so that research on bacteriology could be conducted there.[33] The Chamber of Commerce appointed a committee to evaluate the quarantine situation. The committee consisted of Drs. Stephen Smith, Abraham Jacobi, E. G. Janeway, T. Mitchell Prudden, Richard Derby, Hermann Biggs, and Alan McLane Hamilton, all members of the Committee of Conference of the New York Academy of Medicine. With two exceptions, the members of this committee were the very physicians who had severed their connections with the Health Department in June.

The management of the quarantine was garnering a good deal of public attention. On September 3, two more ships arrived from Hamburg, both reporting deaths at sea from "cholerine."[34] The Board of Health's president, Charles Wilson, daily assured the city that the health officer of the port, Dr. William Jenkins, had everything under control. But to protect the department's reputation, Wilson made sure that other prominent physicians reviewed the work on the islands in the harbor. As the efficacy of quarantine declined, William Henry Welch received an urgent telegram from Jenkins, requesting help. Welch made a hasty visit to New York, where he urged Jenkins to bring in Prudden and follow his advice.

In the midst of growing public fear of cholera, hospitals were readied, extra physicians sworn in to conduct house-to-house inspections, and ships of the United States Navy prepared to enforce a twenty-day quarantine. Each day, the *New York Times* reported these activities as front-page news. The city assured the Health Department that all necessary funds would be made available. On September 9, the steamship *Scandia* arrived in New York from Hamburg, with another thirty-two deaths reported at sea. The same day, Bryant went before the Board of Estimate requesting funding for a new division of bacteriology and disinfection, with Hermann Biggs as its head. The request was immediately granted; the New York Health Department announced the creation of a Division of Pathology, Bacteriology, and Disinfection, under Biggs's direction. On September 15, Charles Wilson invited the New York Academy of Medicine's committee to evaluate the preparations within the city for the treatment of cholera and to suggest measures to prevent the spread of the disease. On the same day, T. Mitchell Prudden was reappointed to a consulting position in the Health Department, specifically to consult with Biggs on the organization of the new division.[35]

Biggs was already doing bacteriological examinations for the city Health Department from his position at the Carnegie Laboratory; now he would carry on much the same work, but with the aid of nine medical inspectors and sixteen disinfectors who would act on his diagnoses.[36] The Health Department did not allocate new funds for the bacteriological laboratory until April 1893; it took another three years until the division was given well-equipped quarters and a properly qualified staff. In the meantime, Biggs performed his tests at the Carnegie Laboratory and had others conducted for him by William H. Park at the laboratory of Columbia's College of Physicians and Surgeons and by his cousin, George Biggs, a pathologist at the New York Hospital. When a case of cholera was confirmed in the laboratory, a Health Department crew was dispatched to the patient's home, the lodgings scrubbed and fumigated, water pipes flushed with disinfectant, and all clothes and bedding removed to be treated or cremated. During the threatened epidemic of 1892, Biggs examined twenty-four suspicious cases. He identified twelve of them as Asiatic cholera, being careful to have his laboratory diagnoses checked by Prudden, Welch, and other prominent bacteriologists who could confirm his findings.

To everyone's relief, no general outbreak of cholera occurred. Board president

Wilson claimed that the Health Department had done everything possible to protect the city's population from any current or future threat of cholera: "All that science can do, has been done in the way of preparation should the pest come; all that science can suggest to lessen the evil effects of the pest, should it break out, is either finished or now in the course of completion."[37] Wilson declared the new Division of Pathology, Bacteriology, and Disinfection a permanent safeguard against cholera; it was also a necessary safeguard against criticism that he, as a layman, was improperly swayed by political considerations and insufficiently attentive to the latest medical and scientific knowledge. Wilson was delighted that, under his leadership, New York City had been more successful than Hamburg in using modern, scientific methods to prevent cholera.

The political role of the bacteriological laboratory was probably more important than any specific scientific contributions during the cholera scare of 1892. David Blancher argues that the laboratory diagnoses deserve little credit for the absence of an epidemic, since identification of the disease, fumigation, and disinfection were all carried out after the period of greatest contamination had passed.[38] Whatever the reality, Hermann Biggs was quick to claim full credit for fending off the threatened epidemic on behalf of the Health Department and his bacteriological laboratory. He declared that the bacteriological examinations had been crucial to protecting the health of the city, and he also gave the Health Department credit for the rapid disinfection of houses and property and for the cleanliness of water and food supplies.[39] The *New York Times* reported that the city's cleaner streets and tenements had protected the population from disaster.[40] Perhaps it was lucky accident that New York avoided cholera in 1892; perhaps it was due to the imposition of stricter quarantine regulations. We cannot be certain of the reasons. What is clear, however, is that Hermann Biggs did not lose an opportunity to promote the cause of public health in general and bacteriology in particular. With an exquisite sense of political timing, Biggs turned the absence of disaster into a triumph of public relations. Relieved of the fear of cholera, New York's citizens were happy to applaud the Health Department.

The threat of cholera to New York did not end with the scare of 1892. During the summer of 1893, reports of cholera outbreaks reappeared in the popular press, and New Yorkers were reminded of their vulnerability to disease in the nation's busiest port. Some directly blamed immigrants. As George Shrady, editor of the *Medical Record*, bluntly stated in January 1893, "Immigration is accountable for the introduction of cholera into this country."[41] This continuing threat of cholera guaranteed the survival of Biggs's new division. The same George Shrady declared that the bacteriological work of Biggs and Prudden had saved the city from cholera in both 1887 and 1892.[42]

By enlisting physicians in the anticholera effort, the Health Department had partially healed the breach of the summer of 1892. Although the Medical Advisory Board was not reestablished until 1899, some physicians were reassured that the Health Department would continue to seek the advice of leaders of the medical profession. Others, however, were skeptical that the department could ever remain above political influence. T. Mitchell Prudden, for example, came out of the summer scandal and the cholera scare with a renewed determination that the country needed a National Bureau of Health, staffed with trained and experienced men, not with (as he unkindly described some members of the Health Department) "the flotsam and jetsam of the political ocean, from which too often strange, uncouth things are stranded in offices where malfeasance may mean death to some, disease to many."[43] In Prudden's view, only the national government could truly protect public health interests from the interference of local politics. Hermann Biggs was less pessimistic. Having triumphed from a political crisis in 1892, Biggs remained confident that he could use and perhaps manipulate Tammany power for his own ends while keeping its effects at bay within his own division.

The Division of Pathology, Bacteriology, and Disinfection had patronage jobs to dispense in the disinfection unit, which employed relatively untrained persons to disinfect the houses and property of those ill with contagious diseases. At this time, the liberal use of disinfectant still constituted the health department's main strategy for controlling infectious diseases. Biggs, devoted to bacteriology, and perhaps wanting to keep his distance from political appointees, decided that the disinfecting procedures were costly, cumbersome, and relatively ineffective.[44] He managed to get administrative responsibility for disinfection transferred to another unit of the Health Department so that he could concentrate on bacteriology. It is interesting to note that Biggs thought that preventive methods based on bacteriology had an advantage in being less dependent on the collaboration of the general public.[45] Inspection and disinfection of premises usually had to be imposed on a reluctant and "ignorant" public; more scientific and targeted methods would avoid unnecessarily provoking popular anger and Biggs was confident that, when needed, the courts would back him up.[46]

Biggs was more willing to enforce public health regulations in tenement houses than in private homes; he argued, with considerable justification, that private housing posed less of a threat to the public as a whole.[47] It was no doubt also politically sensible to use discretion in enforcing the law in private homes. In any case, the tenements became the major territory for health department activity. In 1890, the 37,000 tenement buildings in New York had housed more than 1,200,000 people, by far the most overcrowded population in the country.[48] At the time, Jacob Riis described a tenement as "generally a brick building from four to six stories high on the street, frequently with a store on the first floor . . . four families occupy each floor, and a set of rooms consists of one or two dark closets, used as bedrooms, with a living room twelve feet by ten feet. The staircase is too often a dark well in the center of the house, and no direct through ventilation is possible, each family being separated from the other by partitions."[49] Health conditions in the tenements were generally abysmal.[50]

Even in the tenements Biggs demonstrated considerable skill in building public support for his programs. Probably for the first time, at least in any American city, the Health Department published educational materials in several languages, Health Department personnel visiting immigrants' homes were accompanied by interpreters, and officials took great care not to generate unnecessary anxiety among immigrant communities by the indiscriminate use of coercive actions.[51] In general, Biggs enforced public health regulations as completely as possible, but tried not to provoke public resistance through bureaucratic insensitivity to local concerns.

Biggs also knew that the successful introduction of bacteriological techniques depended on gaining the cooperation of local physicians. The medical profession was in considerable disarray at the time, with intraprofessional rivalries and hostility between the regular medical profession, the homeopaths, and the eclectics. In addition, the years from 1893 to 1897 were a time of severe economic depression; the growing economic competition between physicians for fee-paying patients was exacerbated by the inability of many patients to afford medical care at all. Physicians were engaged in rivalries with each other, with unlicensed practitioners, with druggists willing to dispense medicines, and with dispensaries offering free care to New York's impoverished population.[52] In this context, any apparent threats to physicians' status or incomes posed by aggressive public health activities were likely to provoke hostile reactions.

With the threat of cholera past, Biggs was not prepared to leave his new laboratory idle until the next epidemic. He now made a critical move that would ensure the continuing importance of the bacteriological laboratory: he turned from dealing with epidemic disease to dealing with endemic infections, beginning with a major killer of children, diphtheria, and with the most widespread and deadly disease of the nineteenth century, tuberculosis. Although the bacteriological laboratory would become involved in testing for various other infectious diseases, its experiences with diphtheria and tuberculosis would be central to the politics of public health in New York, and certainly central to the fame and notoriety of the Health Department in the dramatic decade of the 1890s. Bacteriology would ultimately bring greater power and authority to medicine and public health, but not without a great deal of confrontation and negotiation. Diphtheria would be a story of success for the bacteriological laboratory; tuberculosis would prove more ambiguous and daunting.

DIPHTHERIA AND THE POWER OF THE PRESS

The incidence of diphtheria had risen steadily in New York since the middle of the nineteenth century; 1894 had been a peak year, with almost 2,500 deaths. In the tenement districts of the city, local epidemics were frequent and commonplace. Along East 110th Street, for example, in the heavily populated Italian district, each house in the block had at least one case of diphtheria, and some houses had fifteen to twenty cases.[53] Diphtheria was all the more distressing because it attacked young children, causing rapid and painful death, and because physicians had long been frustrated in their efforts to treat or control the disease.

The clinical diagnosis of diphtheria posed considerable problems. Physicians could barely distinguish mild cases from other throat ailments. Several infections, including scarlet fever and strep throat, could produce symptoms that looked very much like diphtheria. Only the most severe life-threatening cases could be diagnosed with certainty. Furthermore, the available treatments produced few consistent results. The problem, so intractable to clinicians, seemed by 1890 to be amenable to bacteriological diagnosis; it therefore served Biggs's goal of demonstrating the importance of the bacteriological laboratory to the public, the physicians, and the politicians of New York.

In the 1880s, Klebs and Loeffler had described a bacillus associated with clinical diphtheria. By 1890, further clinical and bacteriological studies had confirmed that the Klebs-Loeffler bacillus was responsible for the disease and could be used as a method of positive diagnosis. American researchers, including T. Mitchell Prudden, were still unconvinced by the German work, and in 1890 Prudden offered William Hallock Park a scholarship at Columbia to study the problem. At this point, Park's only training in bacteriology was a two-week course he had taken while a medical student; after two years of work in Prudden's laboratory, he would emerge as a national expert on the disease.

Although bacteriological research had by 1890 identified the bacillus that caused diphtheria, its use as a diagnostic tool was largely unknown to the average physician. During the early 1890s few American physicians had been trained in bacteriology, and fewer still had access to laboratory facilities to conduct such research. Park was the first to demonstrate how bacteriological and clinical evidence could be applied to the study of diphtheria.

Park made two very significant contributions in his first published work on the disease.[54] First, he devised a simple kit, known as a culture kit. A physician could take a swab from the throat of a suspected case of diphtheria, then place the swab in a tube containing a special culture medium that could be examined later in a laboratory for the presence or absence of the Klebs-Loeffler bacillus. The procedure Park developed allowed for a bacteriological diagnosis to be completed in twenty-four hours. After showing physicians how easily a bacteriological diagnosis could be obtained, he went on to describe how it should be used to supplement clinical findings. He made a careful study of 159 cases that had been clinically diagnosed as diphtheria and found that many of them showed no evidence of the Klebs-Loeffler bacillus. He concluded that there were two classes of pseudo-membranous throat inflammations, one caused by the Klebs-Loeffler bacillus and the other by some form of streptococci. He called the cases where no (or very few) of the bacilli could be found "pseudo-" or "false-diphtheria," and those with many bacilli present "true diphtheria." This distinction was an important one: his follow-up study of the cases showed that pseudo-diphtheria, with a mortality of under 6 percent, was far less dangerous than true diphtheria, with a six times greater mortality rate.

Biggs was impressed by Park's studies, and in January 1893 he suggested to the Board of Health that the department employ Park as a special inspector responsible for diagnostic bacteriological examinations of suspected diphtheria cases. Biggs produced the unassailable argument that such a move would save the Health Department money. The department could cut its costs dramatically by more accurate diagnosis; many of the cases being isolated and treated at department expense would prove to be pseudo-diphtheria and the patients could then be sent home.[55] Accurate diagnosis would also save the costs of inspection and disinfection. Biggs estimated that the Board of Health could save half of the budget for diphtheria control simply by expanding the functions of the bacteriological laboratory.

Park was duly appointed bacteriological diagnostician and inspector of diphtheria. Biggs and Park were careful to cultivate the goodwill of the medical profession by offering a free diagnostic service to all physicians in New York. Park supplied swabs and culture tubes to pharmacies throughout the city; every physician received a circular explaining the importance of distinguishing between true and false diphtheria and explaining how he (or she) could obtain the culture tubes and instructions for their use. The culture tubes would be picked up each evening by messenger, taken to the Health Department, and the diagnosis would be ready by noon of the following day. The physician had only to telephone the laboratory to get the results. The new diphtheria diagnostic service would thus use the latest form of communications technology. The Health Department of New York City was the first health agency in the world to officially adopt and provide for bacteriological examinations on such a large scale.

The diagnostic service was entirely free and voluntary. The Health Department emphasized that it wanted physicians to take the material for the cultures themselves. The department's medical inspectors would only take cultures upon request by the attending physician or in cases where the patient was too poor to afford a private physician. Within a few months of the beginning of the diagnostic program, however, physicians began to complain that Health

Department inspectors were taking cultures from private cases. Both regular and homeopathic physicians protested against such "unwarranted interference in private practice."[56] The issue was one of professional status as well as economics. Not all physicians agreed with the Health Department's assertion that bacteriological tests provided the only sure diagnosis of diphtheria. Many worried that the Health Department, by claiming access to superior diagnostic methods, was intruding on one of the most important and sacred aspects of the experienced clinician's skill. The editors of the *British Medical Journal*, while lauding New York's new diagnostic program, worried that, because bacteriological diagnosis was being so generally used in the city, clinical diagnosis was "likely to occupy a less important position than it deserves."[57]

These issues, the usurpation of the role of diagnostician by the Health Department and the potential subordination of clinical diagnosis to bacteriology, emerged as the most problematic aspects of the otherwise successful new diphtheria program. Park continued his studies of diphtheria by largely ignoring these professional concerns. At first, he did all the diphtheria examinations himself; later he was assigned Alfred L. Beebe, a department chemist, to assist him as inspector of bacteriology. Park carried out thousands of examinations and kept careful records, which substantiated his earlier work, showing that the bacteriological examinations accurately distinguished between true and false diphtheria cases.[58]

Park confirmed the finding that the bacillus causing diphtheria persisted in the throats of many patients even after their apparent recovery. It was surprising to find that virulent bacilli could be isolated from a small proportion of otherwise perfectly healthy people who had been in contact with cases of diphtheria. These people were asymptomatic carriers of the disease, fully capable of transmitting the disease to others. Loeffler had earlier found bacteria in healthy children, but Park's studies of carriers were the largest and most systematic ever attempted. He provided the first conclusive confirmation that a carrier state existed in diphtheria. The discovery and confirmation of the carrier state—later personified in the public notoriety of "Typhoid" Mary Mallon—was of major importance both for bacteriology and for the practical control of infectious diseases.[59] Like the best work of the bacteriological laboratory, this fundamental biological knowledge was of clear practical relevance. As soon as he heard of Park's results, Biggs convinced the Health Department that negative cultures must be required before people could be released from hospital or home isolation.

When, however, a laboratory report indicated presence of the bacillus in the absence of clinical symptoms, many physicians balked at the idea that they should report the carrier as a case of diphtheria, thus bringing isolation procedures against a person with no symptoms of disease.[60] In practice, reporting and isolation were enforced against "all cases in boarding houses, hotels, and tenement houses" but not against the wealthier class of patients.[61] Enforcing isolation and disinfection procedures in tenement buildings often meant interfering with the economic livelihood of families engaged in home production. In many cases the police were called in to enforce disinfection in sweatshops for the manufacture of clothing, shoes, or cigars. Health Department policy stated that when a case of infectious disease was found in a family engaged in home manufacture, the work had to be stopped and the goods retained on the premises until the patient was cured and disinfection completed. The department inspectors had to decide if this would create too much hardship on the wage earners in the family and if so, if it was better to remove a sick child, disinfect the premises and goods, and allow work to be resumed, or to leave the child and remove the work materials to a disinfecting station.[62] Clearly, such decisions could be momentous for a family whose subsistence was threatened by disease, and the inspectors may sometimes have put their human sympathies before the strict interpretation of the regulations. If Tammany-appointed inspectors were less than efficient at enforcing the rules, they also helped soften the impact of public health regulations on poor immigrant populations. William Park and Alfred Beebe commented: "[W]e can appreciate the difficulty of exterminating diphtheria from a city like New York. On the one hand we have cases of diphtheria scattered all through the city, many of which are so mild as to be unrecognized, and on the other hand, we have the crowded tenements with their ignorant and shifting population, where proper isolation of the patient from other members of the family, or of the family from other inmates of the building, is usually impossible unless harsher measures are adopted than are now customary."[63]

The difficulties of enforcing isolation and disinfection procedures made the prospect of a cure for diphtheria all the more desirable and urgent. In the summer of 1894, Biggs traveled to Europe, where he reported on the work of the New York Health Department. In Germany he heard about successful trials of diphtheria antitoxin as a potential cure for diphtheria; he cabled Park that toxin production should begin immediately.[64] On his return to New York on August 23, Biggs was to meet with the Board of Health. In an extraordinary move, he turned this meeting into a press conference to explain the new cure for diphtheria. He invited reporters to an "exhibition" of the work being done in Park's laboratory, provided them with statistics on diphtheria incidence in New York, and gave them reassuring accounts of the safety and efficacy of antitoxin treatment.[65] He informed them that the antitoxin would be expensive and could only be manufactured in sufficient quantities to treat the poor if production were undertaken by city or state health authorities.

The papers eagerly picked up the story. On August 24, the *New York Times* enthusiastically endorsed the cure and suggested that "the public will be inclined to insist that this remedy shall be provided and that no consideration of expense should permit the Board of Estimate to obstruct or delay the provision."[66] By August 27, the paper announced the "Sure Cure for Diphtheria," assuring its readers that with antitoxin, diphtheria, "instead of being among the most dreaded diseases with a percentage of fatal results almost unequaled, will be reduced to one of the most ordinary ailments."[67] Over the next few weeks, New York's newspapers continued to report the safety and effectiveness of antitoxin and of Roux's success with serum therapy in Paris, and to call for antitoxin production in America.[68]

Commissioner of Health Cyrus Edson, acting on Biggs's request, now asked the Board of Estimate for twenty-seven thousand dollars to begin antitoxin production. The Board of Estimate refused Edson's request for immediate funding but left open the possibility that the project might be funded later, if "it was shown that scientific work was necessary."[69] The board was to meet again on December 20 to make the final appropriations for the year. Not wanting to lose time, Biggs enlisted the support of T. Mitchell Prudden, now a professor at Columbia University. Prudden promptly paid for the removal of eighty tons of coal from Columbia's coal house so that they would have a stable ready for horses, the animals that yielded the largest quantities of antitoxin.[70] Prudden then bought four horses, began injections of toxin, and in short time had one horse "ripe."[71] Later he presented the horses to the Health Department. As one observer noted, "The Tammany politicians little realized that a college professor was presenting them with a gift worthy of a prince of the royal blood."[72]

Park now began producing diphtheria toxin in the laboratory, and the horses became living factories for the production of antitoxin. The project was expensive. Biggs knew that securing funds from the city was critical if sufficient quantities of antitoxin were to be produced. The issue was how to convince the Board of Estimate to approve the necessary funds. Presenting the case in terms of the scientific merit of the project had failed to win the day. In December 1894, Biggs and the bacteriological laboratory's supporters found a way to present their case by appealing to the larger public though mass-circulation newspapers. This was the first time a public health department had tried to raise money directly from the public through a newspaper appeal; it was also one of the most successful efforts ever recorded of raising money indirectly by bringing public pressure to bear on city officials.

On December 10, 1894, the *New York Herald* launched a public subscription drive to raise the funds to provide antitoxin to the poor; under banner headlines citing the unquestioned efficacy of the serum, the newspaper offered to donate the first thousand dollars to the cause.[73] Throughout the month and for most of the next year, the *Herald* ran story after story on antitoxin. Its articles turned on three themes. The first was the scarcity of antitoxin. The second was its efficacy. The third was the question of who should oversee and control the new remedy.

The *Herald*'s stories created two heroes. One was the antitoxin itself. In the dramatic style of the tabloid press, it proclaimed antitoxin as a miracle drug, unanimously approved by the city's leading physicians. But the *Herald* also created itself as the second hero of the situation—an influential newspaper acting in the public interest to make a wonder drug available to the poorest children in the city.

On the third day of its campaign, the *Herald* announced that it was turning over the administration of the antitoxin campaign funds to an advisory commission composed of physicians, clergymen, and laymen who would cooperate with the appropriate city officials.[74] The advisory commission turned out to be made up largely of physician members of the New York Academy of Medicine. This group then appointed a subcommittee to confer with the Health Department. The subcommittee consisted of Biggs, Park, and Prudden, along with two other physicians. Thus, although the *Herald* had gone to some effort to make it appear that it had sought out the opinions of physicians and other city leaders for advice, the final composition of the advisory board suggests an elaborate show staged by Biggs and his friends.[75] There was really no debate over who would control the production of antitoxin in the city; the funds would simply be channeled to Biggs and the bacteriologists working at the Health Department.

By the middle of December, the stories in the *Herald* began to frame the campaign as a question of "life against dollars" as the newspaper urged New Yorkers to increase their contributions to the fund.[76] Two days before the meeting of the Board of Estimate, Biggs and the advisory board presented their report on antitoxin. Their report reviewed the history and development of the serum and applauded its efficacy and curative value. It presented an emergency situation: the need for the remedy was urgent and the supplies limited—the case for production of antitoxin was clear. The *Herald* promptly declared a medical "emergency," just two days before the Board of Estimate meeting.[77] The "emergency" was at least in part manufactured by the *Herald*, and perhaps by its advisors from the bacteriological laboratory.[78] According to C.-E. A. Winslow, popular excitement about the campaign was fueled by constant press attention: "The plan has taken the community by storm. Rarely—perhaps never before—has a charitable undertaking so completely engaged the best feelings of the best elements of the metropolis."[79] The *Herald* chastised New York's politicians for their lack of support: "It is practically criminal negligence to withhold support to the movement which means so much to the poor," railed one columnist. At the December Board of Estimate meeting, Biggs presented essentially the same request he had made the previous August. This time the funds were approved. The politicians controlling the city's funds had little option but to submit gracefully. The newspaper campaign had transformed antitoxin from an obscure scientific issue into a popular *cause célèbre*.

The bacteriological laboratory moved to more spacious quarters.[80] Besides the increasing demand from physicians for the free diagnostic service, medical inspectors now routinely took cultures of all persons caring for diphtheria cases and all school-aged children in families with diphtheria patients in an effort to detect asymptomatic carriers. Anna W. Williams, a graduate of the Women's Medical College of New York, was appointed assistant bacteriologist and joined Park in full-time research.

Williams was the first of many women to hold positions in the bacteriological laboratory under Park. Both male and female physicians had difficulty developing lucrative practices in New York City, but economic survival was especially hard for women, who were thus eager to supplement their meager incomes with Health Department posts. As the demand for laboratory tests increased, Park continued to hire women for research positions and routine laboratory work. Williams recounts in her autobiography that Park was the subject of many jokes among the male physicians about turning his laboratory into a "harem."[81]

The Health Department made the first supply of diphtheria antitoxin available on January 1, 1895. It was supplied free to all public institutions and to private practitioners for treatment of the poor, on condition that they report their cases. Health Department medical inspectors stood ready to administer free antitoxin to poor patients, and physicians could buy antitoxin for more prosperous patients at pharmacies throughout the city. The price was fixed by the Health Department, and druggists received a 10 percent commission on sales. With the growing demand on the laboratory's services, Biggs increased his staff, including two recent graduates of the College of Physicians and Surgeons, Alexander Lambert and Charles Fitzpatrick, and John S. Billings, Jr., a graduate of the University of Pennsylvania and son of the prominent physician, author, and leader in public medicine John Shaw Billings.[82] Charles Rosenberg has published a fascinating account of the career of the younger Billings, a rather self-indulgent young man and a reluctant convert to the cause of public health.[83] Billings's letters to his wife provide an unofficial view of Health Department activities from the perspective of a disaffected assistant bacteriologist. He reported, for example, on one diphtheria case: "I am tormenting myself over a little diphtheric child I am in charge of—down in the Chinese quarter on Mott Street—one room inhabited by father, mother, grown son, and four children. The first impulse of a civilized being is to rush to the window, throw it up, and sit on the sill, with head outside. . . . Well—no antitoxine has been given so that I could study an untreated case—the child is very ill, it is too late to give the antitoxine now—and do what I may, I can see or think of nothing else but that poor wretched scrawny little atom—I shall never forget it, if it dies. I went down early this morning, fearing to find it dead—but it was alive . . . dimly wondering why *it* should have to bear all that."[84]

There are many indications that the inhabitants of tenement buildings and the poorest of New York City's population sometimes served as "clinical material" for the Health Department. Biggs himself was careful not to stigmatize immigrant groups; little specific information is available about his attitudes toward the poor and largely immigrant population of the city. In the years before 1900, whenever Biggs compared the achievements of public health efforts in New York City with other places, he would note that the dense population of New York and "the character and habits of the foreign-born and tenement population" placed limits on sanitary reform.[85]

Biggs's relationship to Tammany Hall is interesting and deserves to be further explored. In general, he seems to have found a modus vivendi with the Tammany politicians; they exercised patronage in the appointment of the large numbers of medical inspectors employed in the Health Department but did not interfere with the organization of the bacteriological laboratories. Biggs was able to protect his own staff appointments, partly because he had sources of funding independent of City Hall politics. In January 1895 he submitted a bill to the state legislature, authorizing the Health Department to sell its surplus antitoxin. The bill became law on March 26, 1895, with the approval of the governor.[86] This was a brilliant move on Biggs's part; sales of antitoxin generated considerable income for the laboratory and brought it an unprecedented degree of independence from political pressures and budget constraints. For the first time, a city health laboratory had an independent income and could afford to fund its own projects and activities—without waiting for budgetary approval from the politicians.[87]

Biggs's antitoxin bill had been introduced on the heels of the *New York Herald*'s much publicized campaign to build support for the public production of antitoxin. The *Herald* had republished articles from its European edition about the public campaign in Paris, led by *Le Figaro*, to raise funds for an institute where serum could be produced on a large scale. In Germany, Emil von Behring had demanded that the State "take the subject in hand and supply the public with as much serum as may be required."[88] In New York the newspaper campaign had generated a lively public demand for the remedy. Within the Health Department, both President Charles Wilson and Commissioner Cyrus Edson were strong supporters of Biggs's efforts. In March 1895 the newly elected reform mayor of New York City, William Strong, held a public hearing on the antitoxin bill, which had by then passed through the legislative committee.[89] No opposition to the bill was expressed at the mayor's hearing. By January 1895, few physicians in New York had used the serum; none publicly opposed its introduction. Biggs had the mayor, the health commissioner, the president of the Board of Health, the press, and the public on his side, and he also had the tacit support of the medical profession.

PROFESSIONAL AND POLITICAL OPPOSITION

Biggs soon extended the use of diphtheria antitoxin from its original therapeutic purpose to one of disease prevention. He had heard from von Behring that, in Germany, antitoxin had been successfully used in a small number of cases to immunize children against diphtheria. Park promptly inoculated all the children in the New York Infant Asylum with serum he had brought back from Europe in October 1894.[90] Fortunately, the children all survived. Beginning in January 1895, Biggs ordered his inspectors to begin the general use of immunizing injections. The medical staff began to immunize inmates of public institutions and the families and relatives of patients suffering from diphtheria, distributing the serum as widely as they could over the next several years. All this was a rather dangerous procedure, given the inadequate testing of antitoxin on healthy children, but no objections to such "clinical trials" are recorded in the literature.[91] Although physicians could exercise their own restraint and judgment with their private patients, people in the tenement houses were subject to the unquestioned dictates of Health Department physicians.

The most significant objection to antitoxin treatment involved private patients. The first confrontation between the Health Department and local medical practitioners arose in early April 1895 when seventeen-year-old Bertha Valentine of Brooklyn died, following an injection of antitoxin from her physician, James Kortright.[92] The death was widely publicized, an inquest was held, and, although neither the girl's parents nor the coroner blamed the Health Department, the *New York Times* called for a thorough investigation to determine whether the antitoxin was the cause of death.[93] Newspaper coverage of the incident was intense over the next few days. Under the headline "Did Antitoxine Kill Her?" physicians expressed divided opinions on the cause of death. Park, representing the Health Department, tested a vial of antitoxin from the batch that Dr. Kortright had used and found no contamination.[94] Health officials in Brooklyn and New York quickly voiced their belief that Miss Valentine's death was not caused by antitoxin and hastened to assure the public that its use in diphtheria cases was not compromised. Dr. Kortright, however, expressed doubts; he would continue to use antitoxin but "observe the greatest caution. In order that I may not make another mistake, I shall first experiment in every case upon the family cat. I speak now in all seriousness . . . if the cat continues in good health, I will feel safe in giving the antitoxine to the patient."[95]

In the wake of this controversy, the April 4 meeting of the New York Academy of Medicine attracted the largest and most representative audience ever to attend a meeting of that organization.[96] Biggs, Park, and others presented papers on the production of antitoxin and reported favorable results from its use at the Willard Parker Hospital and the New York Infant Asylum. But several of the physicians at the meeting that evening were not so easily convinced. Dr. Joseph Winters, attending physician to the Health Department hospitals, denounced the antitoxin treatment even for diphtheria patients and claimed that the positive results were misleading; some of those treated had never shown clinical signs of diphtheria.[97] He further argued that the medication could damage the kidneys, nervous system, and blood.

Clinical objections to the medication provided fuel to those predisposed to be critical of the bacteriologists and to those hostile to the expanding functions of the Health Department. Some now declared the diagnostic program unreliable and accused inspectors of interfering in private cases. Physicians jealous of their professional status resented the idea that laboratory workers knew better than they how to diagnose and treat patients; the laboratory workers were claiming the superiority of merely technical skills, casting doubt on the knowledge of skilled clinical practitioners, threatening to interfere in the doctor-patient relationship, and perhaps even jeopardizing physicians' incomes. How could laboratory workers, some of whom had never treated patients, dictate to private practitioners that all patients with Klebs-Loeffler bacilli must be treated with antitoxin? Some private practitioners denounced bacteriology as a "cult."[98] Many tried to draw clear lines between those tasks legitimately performed by a health department and those exclusively belonging to private physicians. These boundaries had been clearly drawn in the mid-nineteenth century but had blurred as bacteriologists began to lay claim to diagnosis and treatment. During this controversy, Biggs relied on the influential William Henry Welch to support bacteriology and to counter the arguments brought by disaffected members of the medical profession.[99]

Blancher notes that some of the physicians' complaints were justified.[100] The experimental procedures of the bacteriological laboratory were often rushed and inadequate. Many of the staff had received little training in bacteriology and little preparation for experimental work. Because of inadequate Health Department salaries, most maintained private practices and other jobs in addition to their research work. Their tests were sometimes run on inadequate samples and were dependent on clinical data supplied by others. Billings in one investigation tested twenty-nine people (with only six controls) to determine the effect of antitoxin serum on blood cells. He found that six showed a declining red blood cell count; three were written off as being in the "normal range," and three were unconvincingly rationalized away. The results were ambiguous at best and provided poor evidence for the conclusion that "the antitoxin treatment of diphtheria has no deleterious effects upon the blood corpuscles."[101] The laboratory staff did have specific ideas of what constituted a "proper experiment" with the use of controls, but their application of such methods was often casual and unconvincing—certainly by comparison with any modern understanding of experimental method.

When attending physician Joseph Winters objected to the use of diphtheria antitoxin at the Health Department's Willard Parker Hospital, Park arranged for alternate patients to receive the antitoxin treatment. After six weeks, long after it had become evident that those with the antitoxin treatment were responding better, and only after Winters admitted defeat, the test was ended. Park somewhat cavalierly explained that "although we had lost a few lives by it, we had gained a certainty as to the value of antitoxin which we would not otherwise have obtained, and this enabled us to persuade the members of the medical profession much more rapidly than if we had not carried out the experiments."[102] This was a rather rough way to persuade reluctant members of the medical profession—at least for the unfortunate patients who died and for their families.

The members of the bacteriological laboratories were dedicated to the "selling" of bacteriology and were certainly fortunate that no more major disasters ensued. In fact, the death rate from diphtheria in New York City fell from 15.9 per 10,000 in 1894 to 2.2 per 10,000 by 1912. Much of the fall in mortality was, no doubt, due to diphtheria antitoxin, but the problem of so many carriers in the population meant that outbreaks of diphtheria could not be eliminated unless some way was found to provide a more permanent immunity.[103] Thus, although the mortality rates fell, cases of diphtheria began to rise again in 1900. Only when the Schick test was developed for use in 1913 were health officials able to discern who was and was not immune. Their final success with diphtheria came in 1929 after the development of toxin-antitoxin and the immunizing of nearly three hundred thousand schoolchildren.[104] The introduction of bacteriological diagnosis and antitoxin had done much by 1900 to reduce the death rate from diphtheria, but Biggs's enthusiastic claim that the absolute control of diphtheria was within reach was not yet justified; its fulfillment would require another three decades of work.

MEDICAL "ESPIONAGE" AND THE REPORTING OF TUBERCULOSIS

Almost simultaneously with the diphtheria program, Biggs launched an ambitious new tuberculosis project. Tuberculosis, he asserted, was the most common disease in New York that was both communicable and preventable.[105] In the 1890s, tuberculosis was killing more than six thousand patients per year in the city. Biggs had written about the practical implications of Koch's discovery of the tubercle bacillus in 1882; by 1888, Charles V. Chapin was complaining that little had been done to turn this discovery to the benefit of public health.[106] Biggs, Prudden, and Henry P. Loomis then wrote a quite comprehensive report on tuberculosis arguing for the microbial origin and contagious nature of the disease, stating that it was transmitted by the tubercle bacillus from the sick to the healthy, and was therefore preventable. They recommended the inspection of cattle, public education on the infectiousness of the disease, and the disinfection of all rooms occupied by consumptive patients.[107] Biggs wanted to require the registration of all tuberculosis cases but when Commissioner of Health Joseph Bryant wrote to leading medical practitioners asking for their opinion of the idea, several influential physicians indicated intense opposition, and the proposal was dropped. Bryant did, however, print ten thousand copies of the report, which he distributed around the city.

News now came from Germany that Koch had announced the discovery of a cure for tuberculosis—tuberculin, an extract of tubercle bacilli in glycerin. The announcement would prove a disappointment—as a remedy, tuberculin proved neither safe nor effective. Biggs, however, decided it was time for the Health Department to act and presented a proposal to the Board of Health on November 28, 1893.[108] He recommended that the department begin a program of public education, that all public institutions be required to report the names and addresses of consumptives under their care, that private physicians be requested do the same, and that special hospitals be established for the treatment of tuberculosis. The bacteriological laboratory would provide sputum examinations to assist doctors in diagnosing pulmonary tuberculosis. Biggs's proposals were approved by the Board of Health in December 1893 and applauded by professional medical journals soon after. Not all physicians, however, were persuaded that tuberculosis was a communicable disease. Biggs anticipated great difficulty in obtaining accurate reporting of tuberculosis, in part because so many people carried life insurance policies that specifically excluded the disease.[109] If physicians gave truthful reports of the cause of death, the patients' families could be left destitute.

Perhaps as important as the cost of reporting to patients' families was the cost to the professional status of physicians. Private practitioners saw little benefit to them in reporting cases of tuberculosis and resented the idea of Health Department interference with their patients. When Biggs offered physicians free bacterial diagnosis of sputum samples in return for providing the name, age, sex, and address of each patient and information on the duration of illness, few doctors rushed to take up the offer. In the first year of the service, the Health Department received 512 sputum samples for diagnosis—in a year when there were 4,658 reported deaths from pulmonary tuberculosis and unquestionably many more deaths inaccurately recorded as due to other causes. Most physicians ignored the proffered service; unlike diphtheria, tuberculosis had no cure, so that accurate diagnosis did not immediately help either patient or physician.

Physicians' responses to tuberculosis testing therefore differed sharply from their increasing acceptance of the diphtheria diagnostic service. From the public health point of view, both programs served the same ends: they employed science in the service of accurate diagnosis and were intended to measure the extent of disease in the population, reduce the transmission of infectious disease, and help preserve the health of those not yet exposed to infection. Practicing physicians judged by a different standard: did diagnostic testing help them in their relationships with specific patients? Did it serve the interests of the individual? Diphtheria diagnosis and treatment satisfied both public health and medical criteria and was therefore largely successful; tuberculosis testing satisfied the public health criteria but ran directly counter to the interests of physicians and individual patients. As in much later battles over AIDS testing, the value of an accurate diagnosis to the individual patient was, at best, debatable. Public health opposed individual interests; the battle was joined.

Biggs saw no reason why the practices used to control diphtheria should not be acceptable for the control of tuberculosis, since he viewed both as similarly communicable diseases. But although the view that tuberculosis was communicable was gaining ground among physicians, there was still much debate around the issue. Biggs, who, as usual, had already decided the matter, grew impatient with the slow rate of tuberculosis reporting and was irritated that some physicians still refused to regard the disease as communicable. He assigned an assistant bacteriologist, Arthur Guerard, the task of providing epidemiological and statistical confirmation of the communicability of pulmonary tuberculosis. Guerard conducted a block-by-block study, showing that 42 percent of the deaths from tuberculosis occurred in 5 percent of the city's dwellings: the centers of infection were the tenements and dilapidated slums inhabited by the immigrant poor.[110] On January 11, 1897, Biggs and Prudden wrote to Commissioner of Health Charles Wilson suggesting that the Sanitary Code be amended to include tuberculosis as a communicable disease. The next day, the Board of Health approved the request; one week later it added the requirement that physicians report to the Health Department the name, age, sex, and occupation of every case of pulmonary tuberculosis under their care.[111] Assurance was offered that the Health Department would not interfere with patients in private homes; in the case of patients in lodging houses and tenements, however, health department inspectors would remove infected articles and disinfect the premises after a tuberculosis death.

The response of the medical profession was immediate and intense in opposition to the regulation.[112] The *Medical Record* declared the regulation "offensively dictatorial" and "obnoxious," a clear interference with the private practitioner's relation to his patients.[113] The New York County Medical Society and the editors of the *Journal of the American Medical Association* joined the opposition.[114] Many clinicians resented the idea that laboratory researchers, so removed from the life of patients, should attempt to dictate the diagnosis and treatment of disease.[115] One physician wrote objecting to the interference by "some clever bacteriologist, who is expert with his microscope and test tube, but who has not sufficient knowledge of human nature to secure a living outside the laboratory."[116] Compulsory notification was taken as a declaration of war by the laboratory technicians on the physicians' status and privileges. The New York Academy of Medicine conceded that the disease was communicable and that more effective methods were needed to protect the public, but recommended that the Board of Health delay compulsory notification.[117]

Biggs responded to the criticisms in two talks delivered in late 1897.[118] Rather than conciliate, he went on the offensive and called for an increase in the power of public health authorities, with a central role marked out for the bacteriological laboratory. In return for cooperation, the health department would provide physicians with "the knowledge of the most recent discoveries in regard to the infectious diseases and the means for their restriction, prevention, and cure."[119] Such a promise may well have been taken as offensive and condescending by medical practitioners unwilling to admit that the bacteriologists understood infectious diseases better than did experienced clinicians. A faction of the New York City medical profession now attempted not only to reverse the compulsory reporting of tuberculosis but also to destroy the growing power of the bacteriological laboratory.

In January 1898 a bill formulated by the New York County Medical Society and usually referred to as the Brush Bill, after the Brooklyn senator who took it to the legislature, was placed before New York's state legislature.[120] The bill constituted the greatest threat yet posed to the work of the bacteriological laboratory. It eliminated tuberculosis from the list of reportable diseases and urged an end to the public production of antitoxin on the grounds that "the municipality should not enter into competition with its citizens."[121] Calling for the discontinuation of the production and sale of antitoxins and vaccines, supporters of the bill declared the production and sale of vaccines unwarranted competition with private business interests and an example of creeping socialism.[122] Private laboratories and physicians with a financial interest in them supported the bill, as did medical practitioners who simply wanted to limit the power of the Health Department. The latter group included Joseph Winters, the outspoken critic of diphtheria antitoxin. In general, the press supported Biggs, as did some hospitals, the Central Labor Committee, and the ten largest insurance companies in the country.[123] Biggs pointed out that the Health Department had lowered the price of antitoxin from twelve dollars to one dollar a vial, while keeping the standards of production high.[124] The bill was killed in committee.[125]

The Brush Bill controversy illuminates both the authority that Biggs's division of the Health Department had gained in the years since its inception and the growing opposition among physicians to that authority. Although the bacteriological laboratory's new and radical policies for the control of disease had initially been lauded, the voices of opposition became much stronger as these policies expanded.[126] In the debate over the bill, protesting physicians made thinly veiled attacks on Biggs and Prudden: "The Health Board appears to have relied upon consulting pathologists for advice and guidance. Such men have little or no experience in treating the sick, and are therefore not qualified to give sound advice on broad questions affecting the public welfare."[127] The protesters also took the opportunity to argue that such errors in department policies could not have occurred if a medical man had been president of the Board of Health.

The political support in Albany for these attacks on the Health Department came from Brooklyn's Senator Brush. Brush was not a Tammany man, but he had endorsed Tammany in the defeat of reformer Seth Low for mayor of New York City. A supporter of machine politics, he was aligned in Albany with a faction that felt Tammany was taking too many patronage jobs for its own people; he perhaps had supported the bill as a way to put a check on Tammany appointments.[128]

Biggs, Prudden, and Nathan Straus, who was now president of the Board of Health, launched a campaign against the bill. Prudden wrote unsigned editorials for the city's newspapers attacking the measure and asked physicians in Albany and other doctors, including Edward L. Trudeau, to write letters to the press.[129] With the election of Robert Van Wyck, Tammany had just returned to power in the city and Prudden argued that the whole affair reeked of politics: physicians were lending support to politicians who did not want the Health Department to remain as an independent body. He wrote to Abraham Jacobi who had been a member of the committee of the county medical society that had drafted the bill: "[A]nd it seems such a pity just when the Health Department has fallen into the hands of the unspeakables to give them the chance to say, as they surely will, when the Department has fallen to the level of its leaders as it surely must, that legislative enactments, and the solicitation of this committee and its backers, have tied their hands."[130] On February 2, 1898, Jacobi resigned from the committee and publicly stated his opposition to the bill. The Brush Bill was defeated.

Despite this victory, a series of other events in 1898 seemed to threaten the bacteriological laboratories and the Health Department itself. Tammany's return to power increased the political pressures on the Health Department as numerous Health Department personnel were replaced by those loyal to the Tammany machine.[131] Nathan Straus was forced to resign as president of the Board of Health and was replaced by Michael Murphy, a man with no experience in either medicine or public health. (In 1901, Murphy was replaced by John B. Sexton, a man even less qualified for the position.[132])

In 1899, another bill, the Collier Bill, was introduced in Albany to make it illegal for the Health Department to sell antitoxin or other biological products. This bill, too, failed to pass, and its advocates met with Tammany boss Charles F. Murphy to ask him to issue an order ending sales of the products. Hermann Biggs, however, had treated Murphy for typhoid fever, and on his recovery Murphy remained an admirer of Biggs and a faithful friend of the Health Department.[133] Although Murphy rejected the request to limit the power of the bacteriology laboratory, the attacks alleging commercialism and unfair business competition continued.

Perhaps weary of controversy, and certainly preoccupied with more personal concerns, Biggs now began to devote less of his time to the Health Department. In 1898 he married Frances Richardson; in 1899 they had a daughter and in 1901 a son. To support his new family, Biggs spent more time on his medical practice and less on public health. Medicine was considerably more lucrative, and Biggs was a highly successful practitioner, willing to give much personal attention to his patients. He often complained, however: "I do public health work because I love it and practice medicine because I have to make a living."[134] Biggs had been appointed to the Health Department in 1892 at three thousand dollars per annum; for ten years he had received no salary increase. As he justifiably complained, public health officers were not well compensated, and most were forced to maintain private practices, hospital consultancies, and teaching positions on the side. In 1898, Biggs became professor of therapeutics and clinical practice at the new medical school created by the merger of Bellevue Medical College and New York University.

In 1902, a reform government was elected under Mayor Seth Low, who was "very competent, very dignified—and rather dull," at least in comparison with his Tammany predecessors.[135] Ernst J. Lederle was appointed health commissioner, and Hermann Biggs was given the post of "general medical officer" in which he would be involved in major decisions but be free of administrative burdens. Under the new administration, Lederle proceeded to reform the Health Department and weed out personnel appointed during the Tammany administrations. Many of these people were no doubt inefficient, if they worked at all.

Despite the inefficiency and political influence, the Tammany administrations had provided a relatively comfortable environment for Biggs's ambitions. John Duffy notes that S. Josephine Baker, the pioneer of child hygiene, found Tammany politicians easier to get along with than the reform administrations.[136] Baker said that the department benefited from the same factors that accounted for Tammany's hold on the people: "large spending and innate humanity."[137]

In any case, Seth Low's reform administration brought new problems to the bacteriological laboratories. In 1902, a delegation of druggists and manufacturing chemists visited Mayor Low to urge him to stop the Health Department from selling vaccine virus and antitoxin.[138] The delegates carried a petition, signed by over one thousand physicians and manufacturing wholesale and retail druggists, attacking the department's "commercialism."[139] Under the reform administration, the conservative physicians and druggists accomplished what they had earlier attempted and failed to achieve during the Tammany administrations. In 1902, Commissioner of Health Ernst J. Lederle announced that private companies were manufacturing high-quality antitoxin and, with this justification, recommended to the mayor that the Health Department stop selling antitoxin outside New York City.[140] This decision effectively undercut the power of the bacteriology laboratory and endangered its budget, because salaries in the division were paid out of the funds raised by the sales of biological products. Soon, other cities were begging the Health Department to resume production and sale of the antitoxin because of the high price of antitoxin produced by the private commercial laboratories.[141]

In 1903, Seth Low lost the mayoral election, Tammany again returned to power, and Lederle was pushed out of the Health Department. He quickly arranged capital backing for a business devoted to chemical and bacteriological analysis. He took with him several members of the New York Health Department and incorporated the Lederle Antitoxin Laboratories. The Lederle Laboratories supplied the same high standard of antitoxin that had been produced by the New York City Health Department and sold it to city health departments in Chicago and Philadelphia, and state boards of health in Ohio, Minnesota, Kentucky, Maryland, Illinois, and Rhode Island.[142] The Lederle Laboratories would become one of the country's most successful pharmaceutical companies, employing well-trained scientists, and producing antitoxin and other biological products for a growing market. Jonathan Liebenau argues that commercial pharmaceutical manufacturers learned what they could from public health departments, lured personnel away from municipal laboratories, and then fought to reduce the public production of pharmaceutical products.[143] This both eliminated an important source of income for health departments and contributed to the dramatic expansion of the pharmaceutical industry.[144]

THE RECIPE FOR SUCCESS: SCIENCE AND POLITICS

The contributions of Hermann Biggs, William Park, and their co-workers had demonstrated the immense practical usefulness of a city health department laboratory. As the department staff expanded, Park acted as general manager of the scientific activities of the laboratory while Biggs acted as propagandist and public defender. In terms of the national impact of the New York bacteriological laboratory, Park's detailed, painstaking, scientific work was, of course, at the heart of the laboratory's fame and purpose; but it was Biggs who publicized its programs and spread the gospel of applying the new scientific knowledge to public health. The laboratory probably would not have survived and certainly would not have gained its major reputation for innovation had it not been for Biggs's ability to present and promote its programs to politicians, physicians, journalists, and the general public. The preeminent role of New York's Health Department was, to a very large degree, the product of Hermann Biggs's brilliance at public relations. Park and Biggs thus played different roles in the bacteriological laboratory in accord with their personalities and temperaments. Park had the patience and devotion to detail that practical laboratory work demanded; Biggs had the flair for publicity and the political instincts that proved essential to the laboratory's success.

Biggs had the ability to sense political opportunity and to seize the moment; to profit from success and also from crisis. When the department was mired in scandal in 1892 and most of the leading physicians were resigning their posts, Biggs stayed; he was there, centrally positioned in a weak and threatened organization, to deal with cholera when it arrived a few months later. Biggs emerged from this crisis a public health hero, head of the new Division of Bacteriology he had long desired. As we have seen, Biggs had few impulses to modest self-effacement; he made sure that his laboratory gained much of the credit for having saved New York City from cholera. He used this triumph as a starting point for other campaigns—most successfully against diphtheria in promoting bacteriological diagnosis and the use of antitoxin for the treatment and prevention of disease. Biggs was extraordinarily effective in using the press and public opinion to build a supportive base for Health Department programs; he was perhaps the first, and certainly the most successful, public health leader to use the media to promote the public's health. Biggs was also extremely talented in dealing with the intricacies of New York City politics; for the most part, he was able to work with professional leaders and political appointees, with machine pols and reformers alike. He knew how to trade favors and how to shield his key people from political interference. He was judicious in the use of limited funds and imaginative in finding new ways of making money—and he retained the profits from pharmaceutical production to pay the salaries of scientific workers. Over and over again, he took risks, and for the most part, they paid off. Much of the New York bacteriological laboratory's reputation and success resulted from Biggs's willingness to take bacteriological knowledge that was then somewhat speculative and apply it aggressively. Where others might have moved more cautiously, Biggs rarely hesitated.

In his public statements, Biggs admitted to no doubts about the scientific knowledge he used to justify his activities. He displayed complete confidence in the rightness of his actions, ignored any ambiguities, and minimized all problems. He believed passionately in the value of the new science and in the moral imperative to put that knowledge into practice. In this aspect at least, he was true to the traditions of progressive reform. Biggs used his political skills and his social connections to sell politicians and the public on the value of science, and in turn he used science to promote his own political and adminis-trative career in public health.

Despite the bruising battles with a medical profession concerned about pro-tecting its patient base, Biggs's bacteriological laboratory was an undoubted success. Within ten years, New York's Health Department had gained a na-tional and international reputation—largely due to the activities and programs of its bacteriological division. Within a few years of the establishment of the New York laboratory, similar ones were set up in Massachusetts, Philadelphia, and other large cities across the country.[145] Public health officers from almost every state came to New York for instruction in laboratory diagnostic techniques. State and local diagnostic laboratories followed New York City by expanding their programs in infectious disease control.

A major and continuing problem for the New York laboratory was the annual struggle over the budget. As immigrant populations continued to increase dramatically, an ever larger proportion of the city's budget was channeled into basic services, with little additional funding available for bacteriological research. With research perceived as an optional "extra" activity, it was especially difficult for the bacteriological laboratory to lose the essential financial cushion provided by the sales of antitoxin and other biological products. When these internal funds were reduced, the laboratory also lost some of its independence. In the 1890s, the bacteriological laboratories had dominated the activities of the department in both scientific importance and public impact. In the 1900s and 1910s, however, the most rapidly developing areas of Health Department activity tended to be public health nursing, child hygiene and the reduction of infant mortality, school health inspections, the care of tuberculosis patients, and the construction of tuberculosis hospitals.[146]

In 1913 Hermann Biggs retired from the Health Department; in 1914 he became commissioner of health of New York State. In his letter of resignation to Ernst J. Lederle, now reappointed city commissioner of health for a second term, Biggs summarized the accomplishments of the Health Department during the twenty-six years when he had been its dominant force. He took the opportunity to claim well-deserved credit for aggressive and innovative public health leadership:

> I do not believe the citizens of New York fully realize how far in advance of most of the great cities of the world our administration of the health service has been. During frequent trips to Europe in the last twenty years, I have made a careful study of the work of the health authorities in Great Britain, France, and Germany, and have been greatly impressed with the fact that they were slowly, and often very incompletely, adopting the measures which have proved most successful here. This fact has been long recognized in Europe and the authorities there constantly look to New York for suggestions and directions in new methods in sanitary work.[147]

Biggs went on to state that the death rate in New York had been reduced by half within twenty-five years, from about 26 per thousand in 1888 to about 13.8 per thousand in 1913—a saving of some 65,000 lives. Although Biggs admitted that the reduction in the death rate could not be solely attributed to the activities of the health department, he claimed that it was "by far the largest single factor, and in my judgment, more influential, than all the others combined."[148] Biggs was not a man given to excess modesty, but few would wish to deny him some significant credit for the improvement of the health and the extension of life expectancy of New Yorkers. About one-tenth of the fall in overall mortality rates was due to a dramatic decline in deaths from diphtheria. Other department activities had no doubt contributed to reductions in infectious diseases such as typhoid fever and infant diarrhea.[149] Biggs's energy, intelligence, and dedication had helped make the New York Health Department a model, nationally and internationally, of effective public health organization.

The accomplishments of the New York bacteriological laboratory led many other state and municipal health departments to try to emulate its example.[150] The therapeutic and financial success of diphtheria antitoxin led to the production of other serum therapies and vaccines; laboratories began to make or distribute smallpox vaccine and other biologicals. Bacteriological laboratories, however, were often caught between the hostility of the medical profession who wanted to reduce their power and the parsimony of city councils and taxpayers who were reluctant to spend money for research and provided only minimal salaries.[151]

The attack on the "commercialism" of municipal laboratories producing their own biological products reduced the one opportunity they had of funding their activities with some degree of independence from city budgets. Many would be confined to relatively routine testing and service operations without the freedom to engage in exploratory research. In the future, commercial pharmaceutical companies would take over the production of biologicals for sale, and also absorb the profits to be derived from such activity. Also in the future, clinical laboratories affiliated with·teaching hospitals and universities would be more successful than municipal health departments at promoting and funding research activities.[152] The leader of research in New York after 1904 would be the well-endowed Rockefeller Institute for Medical Research.[153]

In New York City, however, the bacteriological laboratory held its own under Park's leadership. The outstanding reputation of the laboratory and of its research scientists meant that Park was able to obtain significant funding from private foundations and university grants to support cutting-edge research, which continued well into the 1930s.[154] It would, of course, prove difficult to sustain the excitement, energy, and creativity of the bacteriology laboratory under the leadership of Biggs and Park in the 1890s. Their successes helped bring about the triumph of bacteriology in medicine in a context where the fight against "Bacillus politicus," in Mayor Fiorello La Guardia's memorable phrase, was as important as their fight against disease.[155] Biggs had helped reduce the influence of politics by his own mastery of the political process, the media, and public relations; in doing so, he helped provided a context in which science could flourish and the public health be well served.

Notes

The authors would like to thank Theodore M. Brown, Bert Hansen, Nancy Krieger, Harry Marks, and David Rosner for their comments and helpful suggestions. We have profited from the work of David Blancher, whose fine dissertation has been an essential source for this essay: David A. Blancher, "Workshops of the Bacteriological Revolution: A History of the Laboratories of the New York City Department of Health, 1892–1912" (Ph.D. diss., City University of New York, 1979). This essay also draws upon Evelynn M. Hammonds, "The Search for Perfect Control: A Social History of Diphtheria" (Ph.D. diss., Harvard University, 1993); interested readers should consult this work for the larger history of diphtheria.

1. Robert Koch to Hermann M. Biggs, May 26, 1901, quoted in Charles-Edward A. Winslow, *The Life of Hermann M. Biggs: Physician and Statesman of the Public Health* (Philadelphia: Lea and Febiger, 1929), 178; see Daniel M. Fox, "Social Policy and City Politics: Tuberculosis Reporting in New York, 1889–1900," *Bulletin of the History of Medicine* 49 (1975): 169–195.

2. Kenneth M. Ludmerer states that "in medical research—as in the rest of science, not to mention the rest of culture and scholarship—America was a colonial outpost, subservient to European direction and leadership." Kenneth M. Ludmerer, "The Medical Schools of New York and the National Enterprise of Biomedical Research, 1850–1987," *Bulletin of the New York Academy of Medicine* 64 (1988): 217.

3. New York's bacteriological laboratories were the most influential but not the first to be established in America. In 1888, J. J. Kinyoun's laboratory at the Marine Hospital on Staten Island conducted diagnostic tests for cholera and other diseases of immigrants. Public health laboratories had already been established in Lawrence, Massachusetts, by William T. Sedgwick; in the Michigan State Health Department by Victor C. Vaughan in 1887; in Providence, Rhode Island, by Charles V. Chapin in 1888. These laboratories were largely directed toward the analysis of food and water. See James H. Cassedy, *Charles V. Chapin and the Public Health Movement* (Cambridge: Harvard University Press, 1972); Barbara G. Rosenkrantz, *Public Health and the State: Changing Views in Massachusetts* (Cambridge: Harvard University Press, 1972); George Rosen, *A History of Public Health* (1958; expanded ed., Baltimore: Johns Hopkins University Press, 1993); Victoria A. Harden, *Inventing the NIH: Federal Biomedical Research Policy, 1887–1937* (Baltimore: Johns Hopkins University Press, 1986). New York City already had chemical laboratories for testing food and water and for evaluating disinfectants and in 1874 had set up a laboratory for preparing smallpox vaccine. By 1891 the Health Department laboratories consisted of two small rooms where chemists analyzed samples of meat, fish, milk, and fruit brought in by sanitary inspectors. See David A. Blancher, "Workshops of the Bacteriological Revolution: A History of the Laboratories of the New York City Department of Health, 1892–1912" (Ph.D. diss., City University of New York, 1979).

4. Hermann M. Biggs, "Preventive Medicine in the City of New York" (Address delivered to the British Medical Association, September 3, 1897). *British Medical Journal* ii (11 September 1897): 629.

5. *New York Times*, September 14, 1892, 2.

6. George Rosen, "Public Health Problems in New York City During the Nineteenth Century," *New York State Journal of Medicine* 50 (1950): 73–78; *Report of the*

Council of Hygiene and Public Health of the Citizen's Association of New York upon the Sanitary Condition of the City (New York: D. Appleton, 1865); George Rosen, "Politics and Public Health in New York City (1838–1842)," *Bulletin of the History of Medicine* 24 (1950): 441–461. See also Rosen, *History of Public Health*.

7. See John H. Griscom, *The Sanitary Condition of the Laboring Population of New York, with Suggestions for Its Improvement* (New York: Harper, 1945); Stephen Smith, *The City That Was* (1911; reprint, New York: Library of the New York Academy of Medicine, 1973). Leona Baumgartner, "One Hundred Years of Health: New York City, 1866–1966," *Bulletin of the New York Academy of Medicine* 45 (June 1969): 555–586.

8. Elizabeth Fee and Steven S. Corey, "Garbage! The History and Politics of Trash in New York City," *Biblion: The Bulletin of the New York Public Library* 3 (1994). For a comprehensive account of the activities of the New York Health Department throughout this period, see John Duffy, *A History of Public Health in New York City, 1866–1966* (New York: Russell Sage Foundation, 1974): 1–70.

9. On germ theory in the American context, see Howard D. Kramer, "The Germ Theory and the Early Public Health Program in the United States," *Bulletin of the History of Medicine* 22 (1948): 233–247.

10. For the announcement of Koch's discovery in the U.S. press, see "Tyndall on Koch's Work. Parasites Found to Transmit Tubercular Disease," *New York Times*, May 3, 1882, 2. For the impact of the discovery, see Patricia P. Gossel, "The Emergence of American Bacteriology, 1875–1900," (Ph.D. diss., The Johns Hopkins University, 1988), 164–204; for earlier attitudes to germ theory see also Phyllis Allen Richmond, "American Attitudes Toward the Germ Theory of Disease (1860–1880)," *Journal of the History of Medicine and Allied Sciences* 9 (1954): 428–454.

11. William H. Welch, "The Evolution of Modern Scientific Laboratories," *Annual Report of the Board of Regents of the Smithsonian Institution* (July 1895): 495–500; Thomas Neville Bonner, *American Doctors and German Universities* (Lincoln: University of Nebraska Press, 1963).

12. Donald Fleming, *William Henry Welch and the Rise of Modern Scientific Medicine* (Boston: Little, Brown, 1954); Lillian E. Prudden, ed., *Biographical Letters and Sketches of T. Mitchell Prudden* (New Haven: Yale University Press, 1927).

13. Simon Flexner and James Thomas Flexner, *William Henry Welch and the Heroic Age of American Medicine* (New York: Viking Press, 1941).

14. Kenneth Ludmerer has called Welch "the J. P. Morgan of the medical community" and notes that "no American before or since has had a greater mastery of the political and economic processes by which support for academic medicine could be marshalled." Ludmerer, "The Medical Schools of New York," 220.

15. See Gossel, "The Emergence of American Bacteriology," 197–200, for details of Koch's bacteriology course. She notes that most of the leading American bacteriologists took this course, including Hermann Biggs, Alexander Abbott, Frederick Novy, and Victor Vaughan, and that they tried to replicate the details of Koch's laboratory organization, equipment, and techniques in their own laboratories.

16. T. Mitchell Prudden, "On Koch's Methods of Studying the Bacteria," *Eighth Annual Report of the State Board of Health of Connecticut* (1885): 227–230; T. Mitchell Prudden, *The Story of Bacteria* (New York: G. P. Putnam's Sons, 1889).

17. Blancher, "Workshops of the Bacteriological Revolution," 21.

18. Alfred L. Loomis, T. Mitchell Prudden, and Hermann M. Biggs, *Report on the Prevention of Pulmonary Tuberculosis* in Winslow, *Biggs*, appendix 2, 393–396.

19. Winslow, *Biggs*, 39–42.

20. Andrew Carnegie, America's leading steel manufacturer, had given fifty thousand dollars to establish the laboratory at Bellevue Medical College. The College had expected William Henry Welch to direct the laboratory, but when Welch left for Johns Hopkins, Biggs, who had been one of Welch's students at Bellevue, was offered and accepted the position. See Winslow, *Biggs*, 268.

21. Ibid., 69; Hermann M. Biggs, "The Etiology of Rabies, and the Method of M. Pasteur for Its Prevention," *Medical News* 48 (April 3, 1886): 384–387.

22. Hermann M. Biggs, "The Diagnostic Value of the Cholera Spirillum as Illustrated by the Investigation of a Case at the New York Quarantine Station. Read before the Society of Bellevue Hospital Alumni, November 2 1887," *New York Medical Journal* 46 (November 12, 1887): 548–549.

23. "Drs. Jacobi and Prudden Quit the Board of Health," *New York Times*, June 25, 1892, 8:1. For popular accounts of Tammany politics, see Alfred Connable and Edward Silberfarb, *Tigers of Tammany* (New York: Holt, Rinehart and Winston, 1967); Lothrop Stoddard, *Master of Manhattan: The Life of Richard Croker* (New York: Longman's Green, 1931); Edward J. Flynn, *You're the Boss* (New York: Viking Press, 1947).

24. *New York Times*, June 26, 1892, 9:7.

25. Smith's remarks and a detailed discussion of this incident may be found in Gordon Atkins, *Health, Housing, and Poverty in New York City, 1865–1898* (Ann Arbor, Mich.: Gordon Atkins, 1947), 252.

26. Ibid., 252.

27. *New York Times*, July 13, 1892, 4:2.

28. *New York Times*, August 13, 1892, 8:4. Also see Atkins, *Health, Housing, and Poverty*, 253, who suggests that since the story of the political attack on the Board of Health did not appear until the middle and end of June and the first week of July, when the Democratic National Convention was in session, the resignations may have been carefully timed to take advantage of this. The editors of the *New York Medical Journal* did print a retraction of the editorial attacking Wilson, saying there were errors in the statistics cited to suggest that the city's health had deteriorated under his leadership. But they held to the central point "that the president of the Board of Health is a politician is perhaps unavoidable. It is nevertheless to be regretted." *New York Medical Journal*, August 27, 1892.

29. The Consulting Medical Board was a Committee of Conference of the New York Academy of Medicine and acted as an advisory board to the Board of Health. The Consulting Medical Board also maintained direct control over the Willard Parker Hospital, which was formally under the jurisdiction of the Board of Health. See Atkins, *Health, Housing, and Poverty*, 253.

30. T. Mitchell Prudden to William Jay Schiefflin, August 12, 1892, Theophil Mitchell Prudden Papers, Manuscripts and Archives, Yale University Library.

31. Letter to the editor, signed "Ignotus," *New York Medical Journal*, July 9, 1892, 49–50.

32. Blancher, "Workshops of the Bacteriological Revolution," 35.

33. Blancher, "Workshops of the Bacteriological Revolution," 37–38, views this as suspect. Biggs was doing his work at the Carnegie Laboratory because the city's laboratory was inadequately equipped. Wilson's announcement that the laboratory was ready for bacteriological research was, at best, premature.

34. *New York Times*, September 3, 1892; Hermann M. Biggs, "History of the Recent Outbreak of Epidemic Cholera in New York," *American Journal of Medical Sciences* 105 (1893): 63–72.

35. *New York Times*, September 15, 1892, 2:3.

36. Hermann M. Biggs, "The Organization, Equipment, and Methods of Work of the Division of Pathology, Bacteriology, and Disinfection of the New York City Health Department," *Transactions of the New York Academy of Medicine* 10 (1893): 303–317.

37. Charles G. Wilson, Walter Wyman, and Cyrus Edson, "The Safeguards Against the Cholera," *North American Review* 321 (October 1892): 491.

38. Blancher, "Workshops of the Bacteriological Revolution," 44.

39. Biggs, "History of the Recent Outbreak of Epidemic Cholera," 63–72.

40. *New York Times*, September 28, 1892, 4. Biggs's views of the importance of bacteriology already conflicted with those of most physicians. As far as the majority of practicing physicians were concerned, clinical examinations were the best method of diagnosing cholera; bacteriological examinations were merely confirmatory.

41. George Shrady, *Medical Record*, January 14, 1893, 48–49.

42. Ibid., 49.

43. T. Mitchell Prudden, "The Public Health: The Duty of the Nation in Guarding It," *Century Magazine* 46 (June 1893), 247.

44. Hermann Biggs, "Preventive Medicine in the City of New York," *British Medical Journal* ii (September 11, 1897): 637.

45. Hermann M. Biggs, "Sanitary Science, the Medical Profession, and the Public," *Medical News* 72 (January 8, 1898): 48–49. In 1893, Emil von Behring had remarked that Koch's work made it possible to concentrate on the study of disease without having to take into account social factors and policies. See George Rosen, "What Is Social Medicine?" *Bulletin of the History of Medicine* 12 (1947): 675–682.

46. Biggs, "Preventive Medicine," 637.

47. Biggs, "Sanitary Science," 48.

48. Madeline Crisci, "Public Health in New York City in the Late Nineteenth Century," 4. This booklet was designed to accompany an exhibit at the National Library of Medicine, September 10–December 28, 1990. History of Medicine Division, National Library of Medicine, Bethesda, Maryland, 1990.

49. Jacob Riis, *How the Other Half Lives* (New York: Charles Scribner's Sons, 1890), 18.

50. See, for example, Deborah Dwork, "Health Conditions of Immigrant Jews on the Lower East Side of New York, 1880–1914," *Medical History* 25 (1981): 1–40.

51. Hermann M. Biggs, *The Administrative Control of Tuberculosis in New York City* (New York: Department of Health, 1909). Biggs's masterful approach to the politics of public health may be compared with the disastrous political mismanagement of an immigrant community as described in Judith Leavitt's discussion of smallpox in Milwaukee. See Judith Walzer Leavitt, "Politics and Public Health: Smallpox in Mil-

waukee, 1894–1895," *Bulletin of the History of Medicine* 50 (1976): 553–568. It is not, however, clear whether Biggs's health education measures were ever evaluated. Nurses commented that Health Department leaflets were not widely read. See Lavinia Dock, "An Experiment in Contagious Nursing," *Charities* 11 (July 4, 1903). Removal of children to public hospitals was considered a severe hardship in the immigrant communities. See Matthias Nicoll, "Requirements of Hospitals for the Treatment of Contagious Diseases," *Proceedings of the National Conference of Charities and Correction* (33rd Annual Meeting, Philadelphia, Pennsylvania, May 9–16, 1906).

52. See Daniel M. Fox, "Social Policy and City Politics: Tuberculosis Reporting in New York, 1889–1900," *Bulletin of the History of Medicine* 49 (1975): 177–180, for a discussion of the fragmentation and internal hostilities dividing the medical profession in the 1890s. Fox emphasizes Biggs's political skills in dealing with the medical profession and in building support for public health programs. See also James Alexander Miller, "The Beginnings of the American Anti-tuberculosis Movement," *American Review of Tuberculosis* 48 (1943): 374–375.

53. William H. Park and Alfred Beebe, "Diphtheria and Pseudo-Diphtheria," *Medical Record* 46 (September 29, 1894): 399.

54. William H. Park, "Diphtheria and Allied Pseudo-Membranous Inflammations. A Clinical and Bacteriological Study," *Medical Record* 42 (July 30 and August 6, 1892): 113–125, 141–147.

55. Hermann M. Biggs, *Report to the New York City Health Department on the Use of Bacteriological Examination for the Diagnosis of Diphtheria* (London: Witherby, 1894).

56. See Dr. Stuyvesant F. Morris, Letter to the Editor, *New York Medical Journal* 27 (November 1893): 666; and Louis Acer, "The First Four Months of Diphtheria Cultures in Brooklyn," *Brooklyn Medical Journal* 9 (1895): 93.

57. Editorial, "Bacteriology and the Prevention of Diphtheria," *British Medical Journal* 10 (November 1894): 1067–1068.

58. William H. Park and Alfred Beebe, "Diphtheria and Pseudo-Diphtheria. A Report to Hermann M. Biggs, M.D., Pathologist and Director of the Bacteriological Laboratory, on the Bacteriological Examination of 5,611 Cases of Suspected Diphtheria, with the Results of Other Investigations on the Diphtheria and Pseudo-Diphtheria Bacillus," *Scientific Bulletin* 1 (1894): 12–54.

59. Asymptomatic carriers of diphtheria are epidemiologically very important in leading to new cases of disease. Diphtheria carriers, however, never did have the same stigma as typhoid carriers—of whom Mary Mallon was perhaps the most notorious and unfortunate case. The fact that there were so many diphtheria carriers would have made it difficult or perhaps impossible to enforce any restrictions on their behavior. Charles Chapin in Providence, Rhode Island, had attempted to enforce restrictions on diphtheria carriers but was unable to do it; see Cassedy, *Charles V. Chapin and the Public Health Movement*, 73.

60. Some New York City physicians cited concerns over the imposition of quarantine on healthy carriers as their chief objection against sending cultures to the health department. They found the regulations unduly harsh, apparently arbitrary, and threatening to their patients' personal liberties; some questioned whether the scientific evidence warranted such rigid measures. In October 1896, in response to physicians'

complaints, and with little fanfare, the New York City Health Board changed its regulations requiring strict quarantine of healthy carriers. See *Journal of the American Medical Association* 27 (October 1896): 774–775.

61. Biggs told the Practitioners Society of New York in October 1893, "The Health Board was determined to make very strong efforts to limit the prevalence of diphtheria in the city, and it had determined to remove a much larger proportion of them than formerly to the hospitals, especially from localities where the apartments were small, the number of children in the house large, where parents were ignorant or negligent, and where it was impossible to do anything in the way of isolation. Patients would be removed forcibly if necessary." *Medical Record* (November 25, 1893): 696. See also Health Department, City of New York, *Annual Report of the Board of Health of the Health Department of the City of New York for the Year Ending December 31, 1896* (New York: Martin B. Brown Company, 1897), 84.

62. Health Department, *Annual Report, 1896*, 85.

63. William H. Park and Alfred Beebe, "Diphtheria and Pseudo-Diphtheria," *Medical Record* 46 (September 29, 1894): 399.

64. William H. Park, "The History of Diphtheria in New York City," *American Journal of Diseases of Children* 42 (1931): 1439–1445.

65. Jean E. Howson, "'Sure Cure for Diphtheria': Medicine and the New York Newspapers in 1894" (Unpublished essay, January 1986). We are grateful to Bert Hansen for bringing this essay to our attention.

66. *New York Times*, August 24, 1894, 4.

67. *New York Times*, August 27, 1894, 9.

68. Ibid.; *New York Times*, September 6, 1894, 4; September 20, 1894, 4; September 23, 1894, 4; September 30, 1894, 4; October 15, 1894, 4.

69. As quoted by Biggs in "Antitoxine in New York," *New York Times*, December 2, 1894, 16.

70. Harry F. Dowling, *Fighting Infection* (Cambridge: Harvard University Press, 1978), 37.

71. Wade W. Oliver, *The Man Who Lived for Tomorrow: A Biography of William Hallock Park* (New York: E. P. Dutton, 1941), 106.

72. Ibid.

73. *New York Herald*, December 10, 1894; *New York Herald*, December 11, 1984.

74. "Anti-toxine Grows in Favor," *New York Herald*, December 13, 1894, 3.

75. The five members of the Advisory Board were Hermann M. Biggs, T. Mitchell Prudden, William H. Park, John S. Thatcher, and John W. Brannan.

76. "Doctors Praise Herald's Efforts," *New York Herald*, December 16, 1894, 4; "The Disease is Always Here," *New York Herald*, December 19, 1894, 5.

77. "Experts on Anti-toxine," *New York Herald*, December 18, 1894.

78. The number of cases of diphtheria in the city during December, while higher than in previous years, had not in fact reached epidemic proportions. Howson, "'Sure Cure,'" 28–31, suggests that the whole *Herald* campaign was the result of a careful public relations strategy worked out by the Health Department. Terra Ziporyn, in *Disease in the Popular American Press: The Case of Diphtheria, Typhoid Fever, and Syphilis, 1870–1920* (New York: Greenwood Press, 1988), notes that beyond reporting the mere existence of a new cure, the newspapers also cited individual failures of the

antitoxin. They discussed the efforts of municipal health boards to manufacture anti-toxin and occasionally attempted theoretical explanations of its mode of action.

79. Winslow, *Biggs*, 113.

80. The bacteriological laboratory had originally been located in limited quarters in the Criminal Court Building. Here, the staff complained of cramped and inadequate quarters. There were also complaints from people coming into the courthouse, who were afraid that they might "catch" something in the building. In January 1895, the Board of Health declared that "there was no danger at all from contagion in the building . . . it was the opinion of the chief medical officers of the board that the bacte-riological and contagious bureaus were not at all dangerous." *New York Times*, January 16, 1895. Apparently the public was not entirely reassured, and the laboratory moved in the summer of 1895.

81. Autobiography of Anna W. Williams, "A Life Time in the Laboratory" (Un-published manuscript, 1936, Anna Wessels Williams Papers, Schlesinger Library, Rad-cliffe College), chapters 15, 16.

82. For the senior Billings, see Fielding Garrison, *John Shaw Billings: A Memoir* (New York: G. P. Putnam's Sons, 1915).

83. Charles E. Rosenberg, "Making It in Urban Medicine: A Career in the Age of Scientific Medicine," *Bulletin of the History of Medicine* 64 (1990): 163–186.

84. John Shaw Billings, Jr., to Katherine Hammond, September 1, 1895, as cited in Rosenberg, "Making It in Urban Medicine," 175.

85. Hermann M. Biggs, "The Health of the City of New York," Wesley Carpenter Lecture of 1895 to the New York Academy of Medicine, *Transactions of the New York Academy of Medicine* 12 (1895): 420.

86. *Laws of the State of New York passed at the 118th Session of the Legislature*, vol 2, part 1 (Albany: James B. Lyon, printer, 1895), 197.

87. *Minutes of the New York City Board of Health*, January 6, 1894, 93.

88. *New York Herald*, November 25, 1894, 5: 3.

89. *New York Times*, March 16, 1895, 5.

90. Park, "The History of Diphtheria in New York City," 1442.

91. The use of vaccines was routine in the case of smallpox where, over the course of many years, they had been tried and tested, criticized, and finally, been judged highly effective. Diphtheria antitoxin, however, was very new and should properly have been regarded as an experimental procedure.

92. *New York Times*, April 1, 1895, 2.

93. Ibid., 4.

94. *New York Times*, April 2, 1895, 13.

95. *New York Times*, April 3, 1895, 6.

96. *New York Times*, April 5, 1895, 5.

97. Joseph Winters, "Society Reports," *Medical Record* 47 (April 20, 1895): 501.

98. Samuel Armstrong, "Objections to the Antitoxine Treatment of Diphtheria," New York Medical Journal, April 13, 1895, 471; "A Critical Analysis of Dr. Winters' Clinical Observations of the Antitoxine Treatment of Diphtheria," *New York Medical Journal*, June 20, 1896, 816.

99. The *New York Times* gave prominent attention to Welch's address to the Asso-ciation of American Physicians in May 1895. Welch is quoted as giving unequivocal

support to the use of antitoxin and the laboratory work that produced it: "The principle conclusion which I would draw from this paper is that our study of the results of treatment of over 7,000 cases of diphtheria by antitoxine demonstrates beyond all reasonable doubt that anti-diphtheritic serum is a specific curative agent for diphtheria, surpassing in its efficacy all other known methods of treatment for this disease. It is the duty of the physician to use it." *New York Times*, October 7, 1895, 5.

100. Blancher, "Workshops of the Bacteriological Revolution."

101. Health Department, *Annual Report, 1896*, 303–307.

102. Park, "The History of Diphtheria in New York City," 1441.

103. Bacteriological diagnosis and the use of antitoxin had no effect on carriers.

104. Park, "The History of Diphtheria in New York City," 1443–1445; William H. Park, M. C. Schroader, and Abraham Zingher, "The Control of Diphtheria," *American Journal of Public Health* 13 (1923): 23–33.

105. Baumgartner, "One Hundred Years of Health," 562.

106. Charles V. Chapin, *What Changes Has the Acceptance of the Germ Theory Made in Measures for the Prevention and Treatment of Consumption?* (Providence, R.I.: Providence Press Company, 1888).

107. Alfred L. Loomis, T. Mitchell Prudden, and Hermann M. Biggs, *Report on the Prevention of Pulmonary Tuberculosis*, in Winslow, *Biggs*, appendix 2, 393–396.

108. Health Department, City of New York, *Annual Report of the Board of Health of the Health Department of the City of New York for the Year ending 1893* (New York: Martin B. Brown Company, 1897), 25–27.

109. Hermann M. Biggs and John H. Huddleston, "The Sanitary Supervision of Tuberculosis as Practiced by the New York City Board of Health," *American Journal of Medical Sciences* 109 (January 1895): 17.

110. Arthur Guerard, "Report on the Distribution of Tuberculosis in New York City," *Annual Report of the New York Board of Health, 1896*, 244–256.

111. *Medical News* 70 (January 23, 1897). The resolution on compulsory notification is reprinted in Winslow, *Biggs*, 143–144.

112. Fox, "Social Policy and City Politics," 169–195.

113. "The Health Board and Compulsory Reports," *Medical Record* 51 (January 23, 1897): 126; "The Health Board and Pulmonary Consumption," *Medical Record* 51 (February 6, 1897): 197–198; "Compulsory Reporting of Cases of Pulmonary Tuberculosis," *Medical Record* 51 (March 27, 1897): 459–460; "A Few Facts Relating to the Non-Contagiousness of Pulmonary Consumption," *Medical News* 70 (February 6, 1897): 215.

114. "Tuberculosis and Health Department Regulations of New York," *Journal of the American Medical Association* 28 (March 27, 1897): 616.

115. For explorations of medical practitioners' resistance to germ theory and fear of the potential of laboratory diagnosis to replace clinical judgement, see John Harley Warner, *The Therapeutic Perspective: Medical Practice, Knowledge, and Identity in America, 1820–1885* (Cambridge: Harvard University Press, 1986), 277–283; William J. Rothstein, *American Physicians in the Nineteenth Century: From Sects to Science* (Baltimore: Johns Hopkins University Press, 1972), 261–281; Russell C. Maulitz, "'Physician versus Bacteriologist': The Ideology of Science in Clinical Medicine," in Morris J. Vogel and Charles E. Rosenberg, eds., *The Therapeutic Revolution: Essays in*

the Social History of American Medicine (Philadelphia: University of Pennsylvania Press, 1979), 91–107.

116. *Medical Record* 51 (February 6, 1897): 197–198.

117. Daniel Fox argues that a compromise was worked out between Hermann Biggs and the medical practitioners by T. Mitchell Prudden and his successor as president of the Academy of Medicine, Edward G. Janeway, which both delayed compulsory notification and made it inevitable. Fox, "Social Policy and City Politics," 169–195.

118. Hermann Biggs, "Sanitary Science, the Medical Profession, and the Public," *Medical News* 72 (January 8, 1898): 44–50. Speech delivered on August 27, 1897, to the New York Academy of Medicine. Biggs also gave the closing address at the annual meeting of the British Medical Association in Montreal on September 3, 1897. See Hermann M. Biggs, "Preventive Medicine in the City of New York," *British Medical Journal* ii (September 11, 1897): 629–638.

119. Biggs, "Sanitary Science," 47.

120. *New York Times*, January 23, 1898, 5; *New York Times*, January 24, 1898, 5.

121. *New York Times*, January 23, 1898, 5.

122. *New York Times*, January 23, 1898, 5; January 24, 1898, 5; January 31, 1898, 6; February 16, 1898, 16.

123. Blancher, "Workshops of the Bacteriological Revolution," 207–208, nn. 42, 44.

124. Duffy, *A History of Public Health in New York City*, 242.

125. Daniel M. Fox states that he was unable to find mention of the battle over the Brush Bill in the *New York Times* and suggests that the accounts of the counterattack noted by Biggs and his biographers was fabricated. "Social Policy and City Politics," 169–195. On January 1, 1898, however, the *New York Times* reported that Nathan Straus was sending the health department's legal counsel to Albany to fight passage of the bill. It is conceivable that Biggs went along. In April 1899, a similar bill, the Collier Bill, came up before the legislature. It, too, was an effort to prevent the sale of antitoxin by the health department. The *New York Times* reported that Biggs testified before the legislature on 2 April 1899. *New York Times*, April 2, 1899.

126. Dr. Arthur M. Jacobus, in his inaugural address to the Medical Society of the County of New York on November 22, 1897, condemned the "autocratic rules and unrestricted and increasing practices of the department . . . including free vaccination and inspection of schoolchildren, regardless of the wealth of their parents or the rights of the family physician; to the ever-increasing control, segregation and free treatment in public institutions and elsewhere of patients suffering from . . . the ordinary infectious diseases, which any physician today is fully competent to quarantine and treat at home, in most instances, and that, too, without the frequently officious visits and criticisms of the Department inspectors or other employees." *Transactions (Minutes) of the Medical Society of the County of New York from November 26, 1894*, vol. 6 (New York: Medical Society of the County of New York, 1898).

127. *New York Times*, January 24, 1898, 5.

128. *New York Tribune*, January 27, 1898.

129. Letters to Richard Derby, Abraham Jacobi, Edward L. Trudeau, January 1898, Theopil Mitchell Prudden Papers, Manuscripts and Archives, Yale University Library. The exchange between Prudden and Jacobi on this issue is especially interesting. Prudden

wrote to Jacobi asking for his assistance in opposing the Brush Bill, unaware that Jacobi had been involved with the very committee that had drawn up the legislation. Prudden was clearly shocked to find Jacobi among the opposition to the Health Department. Jacobi wrote about his feelings on important points in the bill. He called the reporting of tuberculosis "those regulations by which a physician is meant to be a spy on the doings of his neighbor." On the department's sale of antitoxin, he said; "I believe the Health Board should make antitoxin etc., enough for the poor of the city, but not so much for the market." He was opposed to special hospitals for tuberculosis because they "accumulate and intensify the disease." Abraham Jacobi to T. Mitchell Prudden, January 24, 1898. Prudden's reply was emotional: "What you say about espionage is curious and interesting but does this bill help the matter? If the Health Department must let tuberculosis work its ravages unstayed, then certainly, so far as TB is concerned what you term espionage is safely disposed of. But what of diseases in which you sanction this same espionage? Shall there be no notification at all? Shall there be no penalty for the physician who lets his cases of smallpox and typhus et al., take their own way and the devil take the consequences? Isn't espionage per se just as bad in smallpox as it is in tuberculosis? Frankly, I do not understand the point of view." Prudden was deeply disappointed at Jacobi's support of the bill: "I have given a great many of my best hours and much of my best study and thought for more than a decade in securing, in so far as a simple advisor might, just those conditions which are so incomprehensibly—to me—threatened." Prudden to Jacobi, January 26, 1898, Prudden Papers, Yale University.

130. Prudden to Jacobi, January 26, 1898.

131. Duffy notes that the Health Department Annual Reports continued to give glowing accounts of the numbers of inspections made and nuisances abated, but the work was largely routine, the inspections purely nominal, and little was done about any adverse findings. Duffy, *A History of Public Health in New York City*, 245–250.

132. Ibid., 251.

133. Boss Edward J. Flynn called Charles F. Murphy "the best Leader Tammany ever had and one of the wisest political overlords New York ever had." Edward J. Flynn, *You're the Boss* (New York: Viking Press, 1947), 7.

134. Hermann M. Biggs, as quoted in Winslow, *Biggs*, 169.

135. Lothrop Stoddard says that Mayor Seth Low was the "ideal of municipal reformers" who "spoke learnedly and incisively on abstruse subjects like budget-planning and tax rates, in a fashion that moved a polite audience to decorous applause." Lothrop Stoddard, *Master of Manhattan*, 248.

136. Duffy, *A History of Public Health in New York City*, 61.

137. As cited in ibid., 261. See also S. Josephine Baker, *Fighting for Life* (New York: Macmillan, 1939).

138. Oliver, *The Man Who Lived for Tomorrow*, 211.

139. *New York Daily Tribune*, April 18, 1902.

140. Duffy, *A History of Public Health in New York City*, 256.

141. Oliver, *The Man Who Lived for Tomorrow*, 241. The laboratory resumed production of antitoxin and continued to produce and sell antitoxin through the end of the decade.

142. Jonathan Liebenau, *Medical Science and Medical Industry: The Formation of the American Pharmaceutical Industry* (Baltimore: Johns Hopkins University Press, 1987), 100–102.

143. Ibid., 55.

144. Baumgartner, "One Hundred Years of Health," 561; Health Department, City of New York, *Annual Report of the New York Board of Health of the Health Department of the City of New York for the Year Ending December 31, 1903* (New York: Martin B. Brown Company, 1904), 20–25.

145. For Philadelphia, see Jonathan M. Liebenau, "Public Health and the Production and Use of Diphtheria Antitoxin in Philadelphia," *Bulletin of the History of Medicine* 61 (1987): 216–236; for Massachusetts, see Barbara G. Rosenkrantz, *Public Health and the State: Changing Views in Massachusetts, 1842–1936* (Cambridge: Harvard University Press, 1972), 112–127.

146. For a fascinating account of child and maternal health work in the department, see S. Baker, *Fighting for Life*.

147. Hermann M. Biggs to Ernst J. Lederle, December 9, 1913, in Winslow, *Biggs*, 244–246. Biggs goes on to boast that the leaders of public health in Europe had expressed admiration for the work of the New York City Health Department: "Many years ago, Robert Koch, the most eminent bacteriologist of his generation, referred to the campaign for the prevention of tuberculosis which was being waged by the Department of Health, as constituting a model which the authorities of every German city should imitate. Sir Robert Philip of Edinburgh, Doctor Newsholme, Chief Medical Officer of the Local Government Board of England, Professor Gaertner, Professor of Hygiene at the University of Jena, Professor Loeffler, of the University of Greifswald, and many others, after a careful study of the methods employed here, have spoken most enthusiastically of the work that was being done by the Department of Health of New York City." 244.

148. Ibid., 246.

149. We have not attempted to discuss the broader activities of the health department in this brief essay; interested readers should consult Duffy's comprehensive text, *A History of Public Health in New York City*.

150. By 1895, bacteriological laboratories had been established in Brooklyn; Worcester, Massachusetts; Philadelphia; St. Louis; New Orleans; Buffalo; Detroit; Cleveland; Cincinnati; and Kalamazoo, Michigan. "Practical Application of Bacteriology to Health Board Work Regarding Diphtheria," *JAMA* 22 (June 9, 1894): 895–896; Henry W. Bettmann, "Diphtheria: Its Bacterial Diagnosis and Treatment with the Antitoxin," *Medical News* 67 (July 1895): 5. For a detailed account of the activities of public health department laboratories, see Charles V. Chapin, *Municipal Sanitation in the United States* (Providence, R.I.: Snow and Farnham, 1901), 556–601.

151. Barbara Rosenkrantz notes that many physicians preferred to buy antitoxin from pharmaceutical companies than from health departments; the commercial production of antitoxin did not threaten the physician's status. See Barbara Rosenkrantz, "Cart Before Horse: Theory, Practice and Professional Image in American Public Health, 1870–1920," *Journal of the History of Medicine and Allied Sciences* 29 (1974): 71. For the battles over the production of antitoxin in Philadelphia, see Liebenau, "Public Health and the Production and Use of Diphtheria Antitoxin in Philadelphia," 216–236.

152. As Welch noted, however, the state and municipal health department laboratories had served to introduce a more scientific spirit into public health practice. William Henry Welch, *Papers and Addresses* (Baltimore: Johns Hopkins Press, 1920), 1: 617–618; William Henry Welch, "The Evolution of Modern Scientific Laboratories," *Johns Hopkins Hospital Bulletin* 3 (January 1896): 19–24.

153. For the larger context of medical research in New York, see Saul Benison, "A Shared Vision: Creating an Environment for Medical Research in New York," *Bulletin of the New York Academy of Medicine* 64 (1988): 262–279.

154. According to Morris Schaeffer, who worked in Park's laboratory in the 1930s, Park was extremely adept at raising research funds from the private sector including the Milbank Fund, the New York Foundation, the Commonwealth Fund, the Roosevelt Poliomyelitis Gifts, and the Metropolitan Life Insurance Company, and from individuals such as Jeremiah Milbank and Lucius N. Littauer. Park used his position as Chairman of the department of Bacteriology and as the Hermann M. Biggs Professor of Preventive Medicine at the New York University School of Medicine to obtain dual appointments to the University and the Health Department research staff in order to supplement the rather low city salaries. Morris Schaeffer, "William H. Park (1863–1939): His Laboratory and His Legacy," *American Journal of Public Health* 75 (1985): 1296–1302.

155. Ibid., 1300. In the subsequent development of public health, the field of political players would become more crowded and diverse. A Commissioner of Health today must deal with a plethora of community and health-related groups, professional associations, and advocacy organizations—all with many conflicting interests and positions. The job has thus become considerably more complex and probably much more difficult than in Biggs's day.

DANIEL M. FOX

The Politics of Public Health in New York City: Contrasting Styles Since 1920

Most accounts of the history of public health in New York City between the 1920s and the 1980s describe either the decline or the growth of public health activities. Advocates of the hypothesis of decline claim that the enterprise of public health has been less prominent in the life of the city than it was between the 1880s and the First World War, the years dominated by the innovative policies of Hermann M. Biggs and his colleagues.[1] The advocates of the growth hypothesis emphasize that the activities defined as public health and the resources allocated to them increased enormously during these seven decades.[2]

Each of these hypotheses is incomplete. Granted that public health was more prominent on the agenda of the city's political leaders at the turn of the century than it has subsequently been, there is considerable evidence that the enterprise of public health has continued to expand in both size and scope. However, significant changes occurred in the politics of public health while it was declining in salience and attracting increasing resources. These changes made it possible for public health professionals in the city to complain that they were underappreciated even as their authority and appropriations grew.

This essay is an inquiry into the political history of public health in New York City. I want to provide readers with a framework for interpreting what appear to be chaotic and contradictory events. The essay is historical, but it is not strict chronological history. I begin by characterizing the politics of public health in the city since the 1920s. Then I present three political styles that have been employed by the public officials, health professionals, and leaders of voluntary organizations who have been the major participants in the enterprise of public health. I call these styles the politics of accretion, of reform, and of crisis.[3] Each of the three styles is, in the technical language of social science, a descriptive model; an abstraction that is intended to assist readers in interpreting masses of data. Finally, I will briefly explain how the politics of AIDS in New York City in the 1980s was a consequence of the history that produced these three political styles.

Throughout this essay I employ an empirical definition of public health: it is what the people who define its politics and policy say it is. The activities people describe as public health change over time and vary among professionals and interest group leaders at any time. I use the phrase "the enterprise of public health" to encompass the definitions used by influential actors in the history of public health in New York City at particular times during the seven decades discussed in this essay. The enterprise of public health has always been broader than the mandate of the city's Department of Health. The definitions of the enterprise that have been used in the years described in this essay do, however, have two unchanging elements: one is that public health includes whatever influences the health status of populations; the other is that it includes most preventive, many diagnostic, and some therapeutic services for the poor and the medically indigent.

PUBLIC HEALTH IN CITY POLITICS

The importance of public health on the political agenda of city government diminished gradually in the 1920s and very rapidly beginning in the early 1930s. The major cause of this diminution was the increase of public responsibility in other areas of policy. When Hermann M. Biggs began to dominate the policy and politics of public health in New York, in the mid-1880s, the city had no subways, few bridges, no massive public housing projects and hospitals built with the assistance of federal funds, and no responsibility for providing relief to the poor in their own homes. The population of the city was considerably smaller. During the first decade of Biggs's ascendancy, the political city consisted only of Manhattan and the Bronx. The largest influx of immigrants and internal migrants occurred in the decade after 1900. During the city's annual budget negotiating season, aggressive public health leaders competed for resources mainly with counterparts who administered the police, the courts, and public construction.[4]

The diminished importance of public health on the political agenda of city government was evident during the first administration of Mayor Fiorello La Guardia, from 1933 to 1937. The mayor paid attention to public health issues only when they offered an opportunity to bring money and, therefore, jobs to the depressed city economy. He worked hard to obtain federal construction money to build two new public hospitals on what was then called Welfare (now Roosevelt) Island. He paid attention to studies and new services that were paid for with federal funds appropriated for employing the unemployed or allocated under the public health titles of the new Social Security Act. He even scheduled his photo-opportunities involving public health—unlike, say, those involving police or fire services—to display his skill in obtaining federal funds.[5]

The pattern of agenda-setting in city government set in the first La Guardia administration has persisted. Mayors, their aides, and other elected officials have quietly supported increased public health budgets, especially when growth was accompanied by new funds from the state or the federal government. These leaders of general politics only became involved in explicit issues of public health policy during crises, notably an epidemic or the threat of one.

Moreover, the public health enterprise has grown most rapidly outside city government in the past seventy years. This pattern of growth was evident in the 1920s, when the Milbank Memorial Fund financed an expansion of the number and mission of the health centers established a decade earlier by the city's health department. The city's Department of Hospitals, carved out of the Health Department in the late 1920s, distributed increasing amounts of money to assist voluntary hospitals and clinics to serve the poor and the medically indigent. In the early 1930s, voluntary agencies conducted pioneering studies to comprehend the magnitude of chronic disease and its implications for health services.[6]

The most important public health innovation in the city during the 1930s, the founding of the Associated Hospital Service (now called Empire Blue Cross) was the work of voluntary agencies and a sympathetic state government. Blue Cross and, later, commercial health insurance, relieved the city and philanthropic agencies of the cost of routine health care for many low-paid workers and the costs of catastrophic illness for many in the middle classes. When, in the third La Guardia administration, political officials and civic reformers organized the Health Insurance Plan, a prepaid group practice alternative to fee-for-service medicine initially designed to provide physicians' services to city employees, they contracted with Blue Cross to cover hospitalization for its members.[7]

In sum, the salience of public health on the agenda of general politics diminished at the same time that the stakes in public health politics increased. As a result of this double shift, intense competition for resources in public health occurred outside the arenas of public debate. Health politics were not closed politics: no arena of sectoral politics can remain closed for very long in the United States. But key actors in health politics have been more frequently accountable to interest groups alone than their counterparts in transportation, construction, zoning and urban development, public housing, landlord/tenant relationships, or the police, fire, and criminal justice systems.

The provider and professional interest groups to which key actors in public health politics accounted have not been monolithic. There has been considerable conflict among interest groups in health affairs. Within the medical profession, for example, community practitioners who were specialists had different interests from those who were generalists. Similarly, academic and community-based physicians increasingly had conflicting interests (especially after the 1960s); public health physicians have often been at odds with colleagues in other specialties, especially over the boundaries of prevention, diagnosis, and treatment. Members of different professions frequently struggled over matters of public health policy: optometrists and ophthalmologists, for example, disagreed about who should prescribe corrective lenses for the poor and the medically indigent; nurses and social workers claimed professional territory coveted by each other and by some physicians; voluntary hospitals had a large stake in increasing their reimbursement from public funds for the care of the poor, often at the expense of public institutions. Blue Cross insisted on discounted hospital rates in exchange for permitting its subscribers' payments to cross-subsidize treatment for the poor and for enrolling at community rates people who were self-employed or worked in small businesses. Commercial insurance companies resented the discount to Blue Cross. These examples could be multiplied many times.[8]

Moreover, public health politics became so fragmented that it sometimes seemed artificial to talk of an enterprise of public health. In Biggs's time, the city's Health Department struggled with professional interest groups about every issue bearing on the health of populations and medical services for the poor. These struggles occurred mainly within the city, with the occasional involvement of the state legislature. Beginning in the 1930s and with increasing speed after the Second World War, there were new issues, new players, and new arenas. The most significant new issues were modern variants of older themes in public health. For instance, hospital regulation, financing medical care for the poor, and protecting against environmental hazards had once been called hospital visiting, charity care and sanitary inspection. But debates about these traditional issues now occurred in a new, national arena. Moreover, state officials enlarged their role, making broader use of their constitutional authority to determine the institutional governance, expenditures, and tax levies of cities.

Beginning in the 1930s, the federal government replaced philanthropy and state and local government as the major source of funds to construct and renovate hospitals. The federal Hill-Burton Program, named after the act that created it in 1946, standardized the distribution of hospitals and many aspects of their construction. It also strengthened the power of state agencies, whose officials prepared the plans on the basis of which the federal government allocated funds. Hill-Burton transformed public hospital politics in New York City, ending the special relationship that Mayor La Guardia had established with New Deal agencies that supplied funds for construction.[9]

Hill-Burton also encouraged local advocates of expanded medical services for the poor. The federal goverrment, as court cases later concluded, chose not to enforce the standards contained in the Act for supplying care to the poor without charge. But the standards provided a platform for advocacy.[10]

Events in the 1960s and 1970s strengthened the power of the states and the federal government in hospital affairs. Financing hospital and medical care for the poor, a public health responsibility that had earlier been shared by philanthropy and city goverrment, became a high-stakes game with new players beginning in the 1950s. In the early 1950s, national legislation permitted city and state agencies to purchase medical care for the poor from so-called vendors (private and nonprofit providers) using federal welfare funds. A little more than a decade later the Medicare and Medicaid programs made medical care for the poor a lucrative enterprise. Hospitals and clinics that had struggled to balance their budgets with gifts from philanthropists and grants or vendor payments from government could now bill the federal goverrment's financial intermediaries and the state on the basis of fees and negotiated charges. Moreover, the federal goverrment set initial Medicare reimbursement rates generously in order to mollify the physicians and hospitals that had threatened to boycott the program. Teaching hospitals in the city realized that the patients on whom they had traditionally lost money, the elderly and the poor, now provided a greater proportion of their income than patients with Blue Cross or commercial insurance. Medical school faculty members now discovered that their teaching and research patients, whom they had recently treated without charge as a matter of enlightened self-interest, could now generate funds for their institutions and themselves. Not surprisingly, the gap between the earnings of medical faculty and the net incomes of their colleagues in the community narrowed very quickly.

In the early 1960s, the purpose of state hospital policy changed. The purpose now became regulation, especially of soaring hospital costs and payments, rather than increasing the supply of facilities. Blue Cross and the state health department pooled their considerable power in the early 1960s to create an official mechanism to assess requests by hospitals to build, renovate or buy expensive equipment. The mechanism was called "certificate of need." It was implemented by a newly created State Hospital Review and Planning Council. By the late 1960s, the federal government could influence hospital revenues through its power to set rates for Medicare, which accounted for one-quarter to one-half of the income of every hospital in the city. In 1969, New York State government began to set rates for reimbursement to hospitals from Blue Cross, as well as from Medicaid, and to certify the rates hospitals charged to commercial insurers. In this context, city government, itself a major provider of hospital care, often became indistinguishable from other interest groups that were competing to influence state and federal policy.

The politics of health care financing in the United States became extraordinarily complicated in the late 1960s. Skilled practitioners of these politics worked at every level of goverrment, with both nonprofit and commercial insurers, and with a variety of interests in the medical specialties and other health professions. What had been a reasonably narrow set of interests as recently as the 1940s had been fragmented. Before the 1960s, city health officials, a handful of powerful philanthropists and their staffs, and leaders of a few medical societies could define a community's responsibility for providing health care to the poor. By the 1960s, the problems of health care for the poor were beyond the reach of most local actors, even when they coalesced.

Moreover, it was often beyond the comprehension of anyone except experts who devoted their professional lives to the politics of health care financing.

The new politics of race and ethnicity intensified the fragmentation of the politics of health care facilities and financing. During and after the Second World War the black and Hispanic population of New York City increased rapidly. Public health officials and leaders of interest groups became increasingly aware of blacks and Hispanics as recipients of services and as employees, often the lowest-paid employees, of hospitals and other service agencies. The annual reports of the Health Department took little notice of the changing demography of the city until the early 1950s. Then, under a new and vigorous commissioner, Leona Baumgartner, there was swift recognition of the significance of blacks and Hispanics for the politics of public health. This recognition was symbolized by the annual report of the department for 1953. For the first time, one-third of the persons in public relations photographs (seventeen of fifty-two) were recognizably black or Hispanic.[11] In the next several decades, the bitter politics of race and ethnicity could never be ignored in competition for the resources allocated to public health. Beginning in the 1950s, moreover, with the early organizing campaigns for Local 1199, the union that organized workers in voluntary hospitals, the politics of race and ethnicity were often expressed in strikes, demonstrations, and angry confrontations.

Similar fragmentation occurred in environmental policy. Beginning in the 1940s, new agencies became responsible for issues that had long been addressed by public health officials. The city created a department of air pollution control in 1949. Noise abatement was delegated to the traffic authorities. The new distribution of environmental responsibilities in the city was influenced by corresponding changes at the state and federal levels. By the 1980s, many areas of environmental regulation and its politics had become almost totally separated from the politics of public health.

THE LEGACY OF POLITICAL HISTORY

The political history I have summarized had a profound influence on the enterprise of public health in New York City. During most of the past seventy years, and especially after the Second World War, most of the politics of public health has occurred outside the view of the general public, the media, and the elected officials who preside over general-purpose government. Public health has intersected with general politics on relatively few occasions, in comparison with other areas of civic life. These occasions have been, mainly, the financing or opening of new and expensive hospitals and outpatient facilities, Blue Cross requests for increases in its community rates, strikes, demonstrations, scandals and lawsuits, and the threat of epidemics, notably influenza in 1947 and 1976, polio in the 1940s and early 1950s, and AIDS in the 1980s and 1990s.

Few of the instances when public health politics intersected with general politics have resulted in lasting changes in policy or institutional arrangements. Even public health crises have not precipitated institutional change, as they did in the nineteenth century. Biggs succeeded in requiring reluctant physicians to report new cases of tuberculosis because leaders of general politics perceived the high mortality from the disease as a threat to the voters who returned them to office. He was able to make permanent the temporary laboratory he established to manufacture diphtheria antitoxin in 1894 because he persuaded the leaders of general politics that the logic of the new bacteriology made it necessary for the city to provide resources that did not exist in the private sector.

In the twentieth century, however, public health crises have been occasions for visible public management rather than for fundamental changes in policies. There appear to be two reasons for this difference in the effects of crisis. The first is that, in the nineteenth century, proposals for innovation in response to public health crises appeared to have a high probability of success and relatively low costs: report a disease; isolate a contagious person; manufacture an antitoxin. The single best example is the creation of the Health Department itself in response to an epidemic of cholera. In contrast, it has been much more difficult to devise low-cost permanent policies to pay or to limit the costs that result from the cumulative burden of chronic disease (including such chronic infections as venereal disease and AIDS). Strikes and racial tensions are no more preventable or amenable to negotiation and moral principles in health care settings than anywhere else. Scandals are endemic wherever money flows as a result of public policy. Crises led to significant changes in policy only when a vaccine became available, as it did for polio, or for a condition like retrolental fibroplasia (blindness in newborns as a result of the use of medical oxygen), for which an easy remedy was available once the cause was detected. It became difficult even to create and resolve a neighborhood crisis over an isolated victim of diphtheria or scarlet fever after 1943, when, for very good scientific reasons, the Department of Health abandoned the practice of placarding the homes of persons with these diseases.[12]

A second reason that the occasional convergence of public health and general politics has not led to major changes in policy is the changing role of crises in public government. For more than half a century, issues have only received significant attention in general-purpose city government after they have been defined as crises. Creating credible crises has become the best way for officials or interest groups to escalate an issue on a crowded city political agenda. Political leaders define their purpose in managing a crisis as making it recede with the maximum credit to themselves and the minimum memorable harm to substantial groups of voters. In a political environment in which most crises are made by clever people who are angry or upset, it is highly practical to define success in crisis-management as some combination of reallocating resources and obtaining favorable attention from the media.

Since creating a crisis is at best only temporarily effective in raising the salience of issues on the agenda of city politics, leaders of the public health enterprise have devised other political styles to achieve their goals. One style I call the politics of accretion; the other the politics of reform. Taken together, these three political styles—crisis, accretion, and reform—have provided leaders in the public health enterprise with an arsenal of political weapons.

As I present them, the three styles are descriptive models; in other words, they are abstractions intended to clarify masses of data. Leaders of the public health enterprise have not chosen to employ a politics of crisis or accretion or reform on any particular day. My argument is simply that most of their behavior since the 1930s can be grouped under one of the three styles, or under some combination of them.

THE POLITICS OF ACCRETION

Accretion has been the most frequent and, in many ways, the most successful political style in the enterprise of public health in New York City. The most skillful adherents of this style have caused a great many resources to be allocated to public health and have vastly expanded the scope of public health practice.

The politics of accretion, its advocates claim, has hardly anything to do with general politics. It is primarily about the use of the best scientific knowledge to measure the illness and health of populations and to implement those measures that reduce the former and improve the latter. A classic description of this style was the remark of one former health commissioner, Mary McLaughlin, talking about another, Leona Baumgartner. "Mayor Wagner gave Leona everything she asked for," Dr. McLaughlin claimed, "and she never had to play politics."[13]

Some advocates of the politics of accretion have believed, like Dr. Mc-Laughlin, that the most important public health policies can be deduced from scientific knowledge; others have been more cynical, using science as a more defensible rationalization for their policy preferences than either ideology or a subjective (or partisan) concern for a particular group of people. All of them, however, insist that the enterprise of public health must expand gradually and steadily. Moreover, they have been less concerned with the organizational structure of the agencies administering the enterprise than with insisting that it is axiomatic that appointments in these agencies be made on the basis of professional criteria rather than the loyalties or demographic imperatives of partisan politics.

The politics of accretion has led to an impressive record of innovations in the enterprise of public health in New York City. Most of these innovations have taken the form of new services or outreach to new populations. Here are a few examples from the hundreds available in the records of the city's Department of Health: public health nurses assigned to domestic relations court (1929); neighborhood clinics and integrated service centers (late 1920s on); maternity and infant care (augmented with federal Social Security funds in 1930s, with funds for armed services dependents in World War II, and with city funds after the war); diagnostic centers for cancer and other diseases (early 1950s); family planning (1940s on); diabetes control (1950s); flouridation of the water supply (1964).

In chronic disease management, accretion occurred mainly outside the city health department until the 1950s. In the mid-1930s, the hospital commissioner, Sigismund S. Goldwater (a former health commissioner, superintendent of Mount Sinai Hospital, and an architect of Blue Cross), collaborating with the Rockefeller Foundation, persuaded the medical schools of Columbia and New York universities to establish research and teaching programs at a new public hospital for patients with chronic diseases. In the 1940s, the Health Department, using federal funds, established programs for crippled children and for cancer prevention.

The politics of accretion also characterized the expansion of governmental responsibilities for the environment. Again, a brief chronological summary: intervention to measure noise levels (1929); expanded sanitarian services (1930s); a study of smoke hazards and other toxins (federal relief funds, 1930s); poison control (1930s and 1940s); and radiation hazard inspection and control (1940s and 1950s).

The practitioners of the politics of accretion often complained that New York City was underspending for public health. In 1933, New York's $.63 per person was less than the $.70 to $1.45 spent by other major cities. Even in 1944, after a decade of La Guardia's reform administration, per capita expenditure for public health in the city had risen to only $.88: less than in Washington, D.C., Boston, Detroit, or Milwaukee, though more than in Philadelphia or Los Angeles.

Other practitioners of the politics of public health used such comparative data to question the effectiveness of accretion as a political style. Even under La Guardia, public health had not been a major priority of city politics. The politics of public health reform was an alternative to the politics of accretion.

THE POLITICS OF REFORM

Practitioners of the politics of reform have, for six decades, called for thoroughgoing changes in the policies that affect the health of the public. Many reformers have, over these decades, begun their advocacy by insisting that a precondition for adequate public health policies is substantial renovation of the system by which health services are organized and paid for in the United States. Almost all of these advocates have insisted that a universal solution to financing health services, usually under a national health insurance program, is an important initial step toward improving the health of the public. In the 1930s, some leading reformers insisted that public provision of old age pensions, what became Social Security, must precede national health insurance: that adequate income made possible better nutrition and housing and thus better health. In the 1940s, reformers supported the various national health programs that were proposed in Congress. In the 1950s, some of them endorsed, as a temporary expedient, a combination of voluntary health insurance, social insurance for the elderly, and welfare benefits for the poor. A decade later, when this expedient became national policy during the Johnson administration, the reformers regarded it as the first installment of an imminent national system of comprehensive health insurance.

The practitioners of the politics of reform also made proposals for thoroughgoing change in New York City. Some of these changes would be in the structure of public agencies; others would alter methods of financing services, especially for the poor. The earliest example of a reformist call for structural change was an appraisal of the city's Department of Health in 1933 by a committee of the American Public Health Association. The committee found that the department "urgently" needed "capable leadership." The department's dire situation demanded "a new philosophy" as well as much more money.[14] In subsequent decades, advocates of reform called for such changes as reorganizing the city's hospitals in a separate public benefit corporation, requiring medical schools and voluntary teaching hospitals to give higher priority to health care for the poor, and creating a superagency to bring better management to the city agencies with responsibility for health and the environment.

The reformist political style was also evident in proposals to change the organization and financing of health services for significant groups of New Yorkers. Many reformers supported the Health Insurance Plan, organized initially for city workers in the third La Guardia administration. In the 1960s, many of them regarded the neighborhood health centers sponsored by the federal antipoverty program as precursors of a future system of prepayment and group practice that was sensitive to the needs of black and Hispanic people.

Many participants in the politics of accretion also supported innovations promoted by the reformers. The three styles of public health politics have not been mutually exclusive. But the priorities of the accretors and the reformers have been different. They were sometimes different as a result of ideology, but more often as a result of who paid whose salaries. It was easier for a medical school faculty member or a labor leader than for a civil servant to be a reformer. At times, moreover, it was possible for both accretors and reformers to practice the politics of crisis, especially the variant of it that emerged in the 1960s.

THE NEW POLITICS OF CRISIS

As I described earlier, the politics of public health crises has had a venerable history in New York City. By the early 1950s, most of the practitioners of the politics of accretion and of reform believed that crises caused by epidemics would no longer occur. "Major epidemics have disappeared," declared Leona Baumgartner in 1966, in an address commemorating "One Hundred Years of Health" in New York City.[15] During the previous decade, public health officials in the city had redefined the concept of crisis to take account of this self-evident new reality. As early as 1955, Baumgartner insisted to the mayor that the importance of the outbreaks of polio earlier in the decade had been exaggerated. She called attention to what she called new "crises" caused by the increasing burden of chronic disease and the explosion in health care costs.[16] Her successors as commissioner of health made similar arguments. Almost all of them talked of crises: but they meant crises of finance and administration that were translated into inadequate access to health services for large numbers of people.

By the late 1960s and early 1970s, the leading practitioners of the politics of accretion believed that the only new crises would be those that alarmed the advocates of the politics of reform. Crises would now result from the burden of chronic illness in an aging population, from growing numbers of poor mothers and children, from the inadequacy of health care for the unemployed and the marginally employed, and from the proliferation of toxic substances in the environment. Many of the public health professionals who preferred to use the politics of accretion applauded the efforts of health officials in the Lindsay administration to gain administrative control of federally subsidized health planning and to bring the techniques of systems analysis to bear on the intractable social and health problems of the city. Their colleagues who preferred the politics of reform insisted that planning and analysis were woefully inadequate substitutes for massive governmental reorganization and the infusion of new money.

The severe fiscal crisis of the second half of the 1970s, which absorbed the attention and the resources of public officials in the city and the states, made it necessary for both accretionists and reformers temporarily to suspend action on their agendas. For a time, there was only a more rudimentary politics of personal and institutional survival. Avoiding retrenchment became the priority of employees in both agencies of the public sector and voluntary organizations dependent on public funds. For a time, the political salience of public health was lower than it had been during the severe economic depression of the early 1930s.

THE EXHAUSTION OF POLITICAL STYLES

The AIDS crisis, first perceived in the early 1980s, initially confounded practitioners of all three of the political styles that had been employed by public health activists in this century. Accretionists had, especially until the late 1980s, very little scientific achievement on which to base their advocacy for additional resources. Reformers had a difficult time convincing themselves that far-reaching change in the organization and financing of services could be achieved with a conservative administration in Washington. Those who believed that change occurred in response to administrative and financial crises made by interest groups were confronted with a crisis caused, unexpectedly, by a virus that was transmitted as a result of human behavior.

People do not easily change political styles that have been serviceable and personally rewarding over many years. Thus it is likely that the 1990s will still be dominated by accretionists insisting that good science should be translated into policy, by reformers hoping that the national mood and therefore the majority coalition will shift in their favor, and by strategists of crisis worrying about how many simultaneous crises general politicians can manage without diminishing the intensity of their concern. As has happened many times before in the history of public health in New York City, the shrewd use of political styles will most likely lead either to what, in retrospect, will appear to be significant changes or to the accretion of responsibilities and resources by the public health enterprise.

Notes

Another version of this article appeared in "Accretion, Reform and Crises: A Theory of Public Health in New York City," *The Yale Journal of Biology and Medicine*, 64 (1991): 455–466.

1. The definitive statement of the hypothesis of decline is John Duffy, *A History of Public Health in New York City, 1866–1966* (New York: Russell Sage Foundation, 1974), chapters 11–12. Duffy claims (297) that the Department of Health went "steadily downhill" after 1918. Duffy, moreover, equates the enterprise of public health in New York with the fortunes of the department throughout his book. Thus the decline of the department was emblematic of the decline of the enterprise.

2. A vigorous and often-quoted statement of the growth hypothesis is Leona Baumgartner, "One Hundred Years of Health: New York City, 1866–1966," *Bulletin of the New York Academy of Medicine* 45, Sec. Series (June 1969): 555–586. She writes (555–556): "Without the ups and downs of (the Board and Department of Health) . . . their eternal vigilance and their willingness to change has meant that millions of persons have continued to live more safely in the potentially hazardous environment of this unique city."

3. Some readers familiar with historiographic debate may wonder why I use the unfamiliar word *accretion* rather than the conventional *increment*. The reason is that it is wrong to juxtapose "incrementalists" and "reformers" in the history of health politics

in New York. Both the accretionist and the reform styles that I describe were incrementalist. New York had a high population of revolutionaries compared to elsewhere in the United States, but they only occasionally surfaced in health politics. The dispute between the accretionist and reform styles was not over whether change should occur in increments or in sudden, revolutionary jumps. It was over whether change should occur by adding services or by changing the structure and financing of public health activities.

4. The rich secondary literature on the history of public health in New York City to 1920 is identified in other essays in this volume.

5. On La Guardia's priorities and tactics see Thomas Kessner, *Fiorello H. La Guardia and the Making of Modern New York* (New York: McGraw-Hill, 1989). My assessment of the mayor's photo opportunities is an unquantified result of examining published and archival photographs.

6. The voluntary sector was, of course, a major actor in public health politics before 1920—especially in matters of hospital care, tuberculosis control, and housing. My point here is simply that the *size* and therefore the political *salience* of the voluntary sector increased after the late 1920s because it absorbed more public funds allocated for health and social services.

7. Daniel M. Fox, "Sharing Governmental Authority: Blue Cross and Hospital Planning in New York City," *Journal of Health Politics, Policy and Law* 16 (Winter 1991): 719–746; D. M. Fox, D. Rosner, R. A. Stevens, "Between Public and Private: A Half Century of Blue Cross Blue Shield in New York City," *Journal of Health Politics, Policy and Law* 16 (Winter 1991): 643–650.

8. There is vast documentation for these points, as there is for the other examples of the effects of events in public health politics in New York City in these years described in this essay. To avoid ponderous notes, I cite sources only for direct quotations or claims that are based on specific documents.

9. For Hill-Burton and health politics in general in these years, see Daniel M. Fox, *Health Policies, Health Politics: The British and American Experience, 1911–1965* (Princeton: Princeton University Press, 1986). On La Guardia's special relationship with New Deal agencies see Kessner, *La Guardia,* chapter 9.

10. On hospitals and the poor and hospital politics in general in these years see Rosemary Stevens, *In Sickness and in Wealth* (New York: Basic Books, 1989).

11. *Report of the Department of Health, City of New York, for the Year 1953.* Municipal Reference Library.

12. The change in Section 89 of the Sanitary Code of the City of New York, which removed the last placarding requirements, is described in correspondence between Commissioner Ernest L. Stebbins and Dr. Arthur Freeborn Chase, president of the New York Academy of Medicine in November, 1943, Papers of the Committee on Public Health Relations, courtesy of the New York Academy of Medicine.

13. Mary McLaughlin, in conversation with author, Stony Brook, New York, sometime in mid-1976.

14. American Public Health Association, *The Public Health Program in New York City: An Appraisal of the Activities of the Department for 1933* (Unpublished, processed, courtesy of the New York Academy of Medicine).

15. Baumgartner, "One Hundred Years of Health," 585.

16. "The Commissioner Reports," *Report of the Department of Health, City of New York for the Years 1955–1956*, 9–15, for Baumgartner's statement that polio "was never a major cause of disease in New York City" and for her use of crisis rhetoric. Correspondence bearing on these issues is in the Baumgartner Papers, Countway Library, Harvard Medical School, Boston. Her successors expanded on the rhetoric of administrative crisis. A notable example, in the Department's *Report* for 1963–64, is Commissioner John R. Philp's statement, "The Health Department is now in crisis, which means that holding the line on the health of the City is in crisis. It is largely a financial matter" (7).

Notes on Contributors

Ronald Bayer is a professor at the Columbia University School of Public Health and is with the HIV Center for Clinical and Behavioral Studies, New York State Psychiatric Institute. For the past several years his work has increasingly centered on the ethical and policy dimensions of the AIDS epidemic. Most recently he has extended his concern to the resurgence of tuberculosis.

Elizabeth Blackmar teaches in the history department at Columbia University. She is the author of *Manhattan for Rent, 1785–1850* (1989) and co-author, with Roy Rosenzweig, of *The Park and the People: A History of Central Park* (1992).

Gretchen A. Condran is an associate professor of sociology at Temple University. She is currently writing a book on the relation between municipal public health activities and the decline in mortality in Philadelphia from 1870 to 1930.

Elizabeth Fee is a professor of history and health policy in The Johns Hopkins School of Hygiene and Public Health, Department of Health Policy and Management. She is author of *Disease and Discovery* (1987), co-editor with Roy M. Acheson of *A History of Education in Public Health* (1991), and co-editor with Daniel M. Fox of *AIDS: The Burdens of History* (1988) and *AIDS: The Making of a Chronic Disease* (1992). She is currently curator of "Garbage! The History and Politics of Trash in New York City," an exhibition at the New York Public Library.

Daniel M. Fox is president of the Milbank Memorial Fund. His most recent book is *Power and Illness: The Failure and Future of American Health Policy* (1993).

Evelynn M. Hammonds is an assistant professor of the history of science in the Program in Science, Technology, and Society at Massachusetts Institute of Technology. Her dissertation, completed in 1993 at Harvard University, is entitled "The Search for Perfect Control: A Social History of Diphtheria."

Alan M. Kraut, professor of history at The American University in Washington, D.C., is interested in immigration and ethnic history and the history of medicine. He is the author of *The Huddled Masses: The Immigrant in American Society, 1880–1921* (1982) and coauthor of *American Refugee Policy and European Jewry, 1933–1945* (1987). He is also editor of *Crusaders and Compromisers* (1983), an anthology of essays on antislavery politics before the Civil War. He has published numerous articles on immigration and ethnicity in both scholarly journals and popular periodicals. His recent book, *Silent Travelers: Germs, Genes, and the "Immigrant Menace,"* has received support from the Rockefeller Foundation, the Smithsonian Institution, and the National Endowment for the Humanities and was published by Basic Books.

Judith Walzer Leavitt is a professor of the history of medicine and history of science, and Evjue-Bascom Professor of Women's Studies at the University of Wisconsin-Madison. Her publications include *The Healthiest City: Milwaukee and the Politics of Health Reform* (1982) and *Brought to Bed: Childbearing in America, 1750–1950* (1986). She is the editor of *Women and Health in America: Historical Readings* (1984) and co-editor, with Ronald L. Numbers, of *Sickness and Health in America: Readings in the History of Medicine and Public Health* (1985). She is finishing a book *"Typhoid Mary": Personal Liberty versus the Public's Health,* to be published by Beacon Press.

Naomi Rogers is a research associate in the history of medicine at Yale University. She has published on the history of American public health, women and medicine, and unorthodox medicine. She is the author of *Dirt and Disease: Polio before FDR* (1992), and is currently working on a study of Sister Elizabeth Kenny, an Australian nurse who transformed polio therapy in America in the 1940s.

David Rosner, editor of this volume, is a professor of history at Baruch College and the CUNY Graduate School. He is also adjunct professor of community medicine at Mount Sinai School of Medicine. He received his doctorate from Harvard University and has been a John Simon Guggenheim Fellow, a Josiah Macy Fellow, and an NEH Fellow at the Hastings Center. In addition, he has held two National Endowment for the Humanities Interpretative Research grants. He has written and co-edited a number of books including *A Once Charitable Enterprise: Hospitals and Health Care in Brooklyn and New York* (1982); *Deadly Dust: Silicosis and the Politics of Occupational Disease in Twentieth Century America* (1991); *Health Care in America* (1979); *Dying for Work* (1987); and *"Slaves of the Depression," Workers' Letters about Life on the Job* (1987). Presently, he is completing (with Gerald Markowitz) a book on race and children in post–World War II New York.

Index

Abbott, Alexander, 186n15
Acosta, Carmen, 98
Acosta, Ismael, 97
acquired immune deficiency syndrome
  (AIDS), 2; and civil liberties issues,
  93, 94, 137, 142; and drug use, 132,
  133, 135, 139, 140; estimates of infection, 140–141; funding crisis for,
  144–147; and HIV testing, 137–139,
  142–143, 177; and the HIV virus, 65,
  132–134; minority groups associated
  with, 17, 65–66, 83, 94, 131, 132,
  133, 135, 140 (*see also* gay community, and AIDS); mortality rate of, 37,
  38 (tab. 3), 132; and the needle program, 141–142, 143, 144; and the
  political process, 94, 197, 203, 208;
  and the poor, 16, 140, 147; prevention
  policy for, 136, 155; and public mistrust of politicians and scientists, 94,
  141, 142; response to, 17, 18, 37, 38;
  and tuberculosis control, 128, 142,
  147; and women, 132–133
ACT-UP. *See* AIDS Coalition to Unleash Power
ADAPT, 143
Addams, Dr. Jonas Smith, 44, 51
Africa and Africans, 65, 104, 131
African Americans. *See* black Americans
AICP. *See* Association for Improving the
  Condition of the Poor
AIDS. *See* acquired immune deficiency
  syndrome
AIDS Coalition to Unleash Power
  (ACT-UP), 141, 143, 144, 145
air quality, 9, 44, 48, 53
American Cancer Society, 121
American Cyanamid Company, 126

American Foundation for AIDS Re-
  search (AmFAR), 144
American Heart Association, 121
American Public Health Association, 4,
  154, 206
American Red Cross, 99
American Women's Voluntary Services,
  99
AmFAR. *See* American Foundation for
  AIDS Research
Anti-Compulsory Vaccination League,
  105, 113n16
anti-Semitism, 77, 87n40, 88n45, 116,
  125
antivaccinationists, 105, 108, 113n16
Associated Hospital Service. *See* Empire
  Blue Cross
Association for Improving the Condition
  of the Poor (AICP), 53, 56, 57, 58, 61,
  110
Association of American Physicians,
  191–192n99
Association of New York. *See* New
  York Citizens' Association
Astor, John Jacob, Jr., 3–4
Australia, changes in mortality rates in,
  27, 39n5

bacteriology, 25, 167, 174, 184; and
  cholera, 158, 160, 188n40; and diphtheria, 165, 166, 167, 175, 176; growing prominence of, 12, 153, 156;
  laboratories in New York City for,
  155-156, 185n3; and public health,
  158, 163, 164; and tuberculosis, 175,
  176, 177–178
Baker, S. Josephine, 180
Bates, Barbara, 87–88n42

bath houses, 136, 137, 138
Baumgartner, Leona, 202, 204, 207,
    208n2, 210n16
Bayer, Ronald, 94, 155
Beebe, Alfred L., 167, 168
Beecher, Catharine, 49
Behring, Emil von, 172, 173, 188n45
Bellevue Medical College, 187n20
Belmont, August, 3–4
Benison, Saul, 84n7, 85n31
Bernecker, Edward M., 97
Bettmann, Otto, 1
Biggs, George, 161
Biggs, Hermann M., 183–184, 186n15,
    197, 198, 200; and bacteriology in
    public health programs, 163–164, 165,
    188n40; bacteriology lab directed by,
    156, 157, 161, 162, 171, 180, 184,
    203; and Carnegie Laboratory, 157–
    158, 187n20, 188n33; and cholera,
    158, 160, 161, 162, 182; as consulting
    pathologist to the health department,
    158, 160, 180; and diphtheria control,
    166, 167, 168, 169, 170, 171, 172–
    174, 175, 177, 182, 190n61, 190n75;
    and polio, 117–118; and public rela-
    tions, 162, 164, 181–182, 188–
    189n51, 189n52; and Tammany Hall,
    160, 163, 172, 179, 180; and tenement
    residents, 163–164, 172; and tuber-
    culosis control, 11, 155, 157–158,
    175–181, 193n117, 193n125, 203; and
    typhoid, 157–158
Billings, John S., Jr., 171, 174
black Americans, 202, 206; and AIDS,
    132, 135, 140, 141, 143, 144
Black and Hispanic Caucus of the City
    Council, 141
Black Leadership Commission on AIDS,
    143, 144
Blackmar, Elizabeth, 8, 25
Blackstone, Sir William, 43–44, 47,
    62n3
Blancher, David, 162
Bleeker, Elizabeth, 49
Blood Products Advisory Committee, 65
Bloomingdale, Lyman G., 78

Blue, Rupert, 72
Blue Cross. *See* Empire Blue Cross
B'nai B'rith, 79
Board of Estimate, 168, 169, 170
Board of Health. *See* Metropolitan Board
    of Health
Brannan, John W., 190n75
Britain, 3, 57, 76, 183
bronchitis, 32
Brooklyn Bureau of Charities, 73
Brooklyn Department of Health, 105,
    113n16
Brush, Senator, 178, 179
Brush Bill, 178–179, 193n125, 193–
    194n129
Bryant, Joseph D., 159, 160, 161, 176
*Bulletin of the New York Academy of
    Medicine*, 144–145

Cambridge (Mass.) Board of Health,
    108–109
Canada, 27, 39n5, 68
cancer, 15, 17–18, 38, 205
Cantor, Eddie, 121
Caribbean Women's Health Association,
    Inc., 83
Carnegie, Andrew, 158, 187n20
Carnegie Laboratory, 157, 161, 187n20,
    188n33
Castle Garden, 68
Center for Infectious Disease, 66
Centers for Disease Control (CDC), 65–
    66, 83, 131–132, 135, 137–138
CDC. *See* Centers for Disease Control
Central Labor Committee, 178
Central Park, 57
Chadwick, Edwin, 42
Chamber of Commerce, 160
Chapin, Charles V., 11, 175, 185n3,
    189n59
Charities and Corrections, 114n25
China, 68
cholera, 3, 10, 25, 30, 36, 37, 39n11, 59,
    68, 75, 157; diagnosis of, 185n3,
    188n40; in 1892, 156, 158, 160–161,
    182, 203; and immigrants, 2, 67, 69,
    162; and mortality, 7, 27, 30, 31 (tab.

1), 32, 40–41n19, 52; and poverty, 2, 7, 25, 30, 32; responses to, 17, 28, 36, 39n11, 48, 153

Cholera Years (Rosenberg), 18, 131

Citizens' Association Council of Hygiene, 58

City Reform Club, 159

Civilian Defense Volunteer Organization, 99

Civil War, 3, 4, 60

College of Physicians, 28

Collier Bill, 179, 193n125

Collins, Dr. Moses, 82

Columbia College of Physicians and Surgeons, 157

Communicable Disease Center, 126

Compas, Dr. Jean Claude, 65

Comprehensive AIDS Resource Emergency Act of 1990, 145–146

Condran, Gretchen A., 25

consumption. *See* tuberculosis

Continental Casualty Company, 122–124

Cox, Herald, 126

croup, mortality rates of, 27, 34 (tab. 2), 35, 40–41n19

Cuomo, Mario, 137, 140, 145

Cutter incident, 126, 127

De Kruif, Paul, 125

Denver, Colorado, 79, 80, 81–82, 89n58

Department of Buildings, 60

Department of Public Health. *See* New York City Health Department

Department of Sanitation, 120

Depression: of 1837–1844, 56; of 1873, 60; of 1893–1897, 164; Great, 119

Derby, Dr. Richard, 160

diarrheal diseases, 25, 28, 32, 67, 156, 184; classification of, 32, 39n8; and mortality, 3, 33, 34 (tab. 2), 38

Dinkins, David, 142–143, 144

diphtheria, 32, 39n11, 184; age-standardized mortality rates of, 32, 34 (tab. 2), 35, 165; antitoxin for, 153, 168–170, 171, 172–175, 182, 184, 190–191n78, 191n91, 191–192n99,

203; and bacteriology, 156, 164, 165, 167, 168; carriers of, 167, 171, 175, 189n59, 192n103; cure for, 176, 191–192n99; diagnosis of, 165–167, 171, 175, 176–177, 182; mortality rates of, 15, 27, 31 (tab. 1), 32, 33, 40–41n19, 165, 175, 184; prevention of, enforced in tenements, 167–168, 190n61; treatment of, 165, 177

disease, 1–5, 18, 43, 61 (*see also* endemic diseases; epidemics; *specific diseases*); chronic, 205, 207; classification and categorization of, 39n8, 40–41n19; decline of, 87–88n42; environmental causes of, 25, 44; and hygiene, 9, 25; and pathogens and bacteria, 9, 11; and poverty, 2, 13, 16, 25, 32, 44, 48, 51, 117, 153; as a social phenomenon, 16–17

disinfection, 161, 162, 163, 166, 167–168, 177, 185n3

doctors. *See* medical profession

Dowdle, Dr. Walter, 66

draft riots, 58, 59

drug use, 17, 144; and AIDS, 132, 133, 135, 139, 140

Duffy, John, 18, 180, 194n131, 208n1

Eaton, Dorman, 61

Edson, Cyrus, 169, 172

education, 37, 73, 93, 176; and AIDS, 83, 137, 140, 143; and cholera, 164, 188–189n51; and the smallpox vaccine, 105, 111

Eisenhower, Dwight, 126

Ellis Island, 1, 68, 69, 70, 72, 83

Emerson, Haven, 71

Emigration Landing Depot, 68

Empire Blue Cross, 199, 200, 201, 202, 205

employment, 16, 51; contractural relations in, 46–48, 59, 62–63n8; and housing, 58, 60; and tuberculosis, 10, 11, 12, 13–14

endemic diseases, 28, 30, 35, 36–37, 164; mortality from, 32, 38

Enders, John, 122, 124–125, 126, 127
environmental controls, 8, 9–11, 14–16,
    45–46, 52, 54, 202. *See also* inspec-
    tion; sewers; street cleaning; water
    supplies
epidemics, 35, 36, 39n8, 207 (*see also*
    disease; *specific diseases*); and age-
    standardized mortality, 32, 33, 34 (tab.
    2); class differences in impact of, 25,
    45; decline of, 36–37, 38; definitions
    of, 17–18, 37; and the housing mar-
    ket, 48–53; and mortality, 3, 7, 25, 27,
    28, 29 (fig. 1), 30, 31 (tab. 1), 32, 35,
    36, 38, 40–41n19; patterns of, 25, 28,
    32; and the political process, 94, 131;
    responses to, 18–19, 28, 29, 30, 33,
    36, 153; social context of, 29, 43, 44;
    in the twentieth century, 17, 37
erysipelas, 34 (tab. 2)
Europe, 75, 100, 168; mortality rates in,
    27, 39n5; polio epidemics in, 70–71;
    public health in, 183, 195n147; scien-
    tific superiority of, 155, 156, 185n2
Ewing, Sanitary Superintendent, 158

favus, 69–70
Fee, Elizabeth, 12, 153
Fish, Hamilton, 3–4
Fishberg, Dr. Maurice, 76, 77, 88n45
Fitzpatrick, Charles, 171
Flake, Floyd, 141
Flexner, Dr. Simon, 73, 84n7
Flynn, Edward J., 194n133
Food and Drug Administration (FDA),
    65, 66, 83
food regulaton, 35, 36
Fourierism, 57
Fox, Daniel M., 153–154, 193n117,
    193n125
Francis, Thomas, 125, 126
Franklin, Benjamin, 104
Friedman, Sam, 135
Friedman, Rabbi William, 79, 81

gay community, and AIDS, 94, 131–
    132, 133–134, 136–137, 138, 139,
    140, 141, 142, 143, 145
gay men. *See* gay community

Gay Men's Health Crisis (GMHC), 135,
    140, 142
German immigrants, 67, 71–72
Germany, 98, 157, 176, 195n147; diph-
    theria antitoxin used in, 168, 172, 173;
    and tuberculosis, 176, 195n147
germ theory, 12–13, 14, 68, 69, 72, 94,
    117, 153, 156
Gibbons, William, 52–53
GMHC. *See* Gay Men's Health Crisis
Goldwater, Sigismund S., 205
gonorrhea. *See* venereal disease
Gossel, Patricia, 156
Gottfried, Richard, 145
Greater New York Hospital Association,
    145
Gregg, Dr. Milton, 73
Griscom, John, 3, 4, 42, 51, 53–56, 57,
    59
Guerard, Arthur, 177

Haitian Coalition on AIDS, 65
Haitians, and AIDS, 65–66, 83, 94, 131,
    133
Hamburg, Margaret, 143–144
Hamilton, Dr. Alan McLane, 160
Hammonds, Evelynn M., 153
Hansen, Alberta, 79
Harlan, John Marshall, 108–109
Hartley, Robert, 57
Hartog, Hendrick, 46
Hatch, Orrin, 145
health, 9, 12, 18 (*see also* public health);
    and accountability, 43–44, 46, 47, 50,
    51, 61–62; and civil liberties, 93, 105,
    107, 109, 177, 189–190n60 (*see also*
    acquired immune deficiency syn-
    drome: and civil liberties issues); as a
    commodity, 43, 47–48; and morality
    in housing, 49, 51, 53, 54; and nui-
    sances, 47, 54; as a personal charac-
    teristic, 42–43, 44, 46, 48, 50; and
    regulation, 44, 45; as a social product,
    43, 46, 61–62
Health Act, 61
Health and Hospitals Corporation, 135,
    138–139, 140, 155
Health Care Finance Agency, 146

health department. *See* New York City Health Department

Health Insurance Plan, 199, 206

health reformers, 42, 51, 57; disease linked to poverty by, 48, 117; environment control by, 45–46, 52, 54; and housing, 25–26, 55, 56, 57, 58, 59, 60–61; and nuisances, 45–46, 54; ordinances proposed by, 45–46

heart disease, 15, 17, 38

Hill, Mary, 73

Hill-Burton Program, 200

Hispanics: and AIDS, 132, 135, 140; and public health, 202, 206; response to needle program of, 141, 143, 144

HIV. *See under* acquired immune deficiency syndrome

Hobby, Oveta Culp, 126

homelessness, 1, 16, 54

Horwitz, Morton, 47

Hosack, David, 104

hospitals, and public health policy, 200–201, 206

housing, 9, 18, 42; and accountability, 47–48, 59–61; codes and regulations in, 14, 43, 53–56, 57, 58–60; differentiation in standards supported by aldermen, 51–52; and the health crisis, 8, 56, 57; and health reformers, 25–26, 43, 54, 55, 56, 57, 58, 59, 60–61; and the labor market, 42, 46–47, 54, 55–56, 58–59; as a market in health, 48, 49–50, 52–53; and mortality, 35, 53–54; and property rights, 26, 45, 46, 55, 59; and public health, 9, 42; and water supply, 52–53

Housing Act of 1901, 60

Howe, Irving, 75

Human Immunodeficiency Virus (HIV). *See under* acquired immune deficiency syndrome

Hylan, Mayor John, 110

immigrants, 2, 68, 158, 168 (*see also specific national groups*); blamed for epidemics, 26, 66, 70, 82–83, 84n7, 86n31, 89n56, 162; and cholera, 2, 67, 69, 160, 162; civil liberties of, 105;

health inspections of, 66–67, 68–70; and mortality, 9, 42, 53–54, 56, 66–67; polio associated with, 115, 116–117, 118, 119, 122, 128; and sanitarium care, 78, 89n56; and tuberculosis, 26, 54, 70, 74–75, 76–77, 78, 89n56

immigration, 9, 56, 66–67

immunization. *See* vaccination

Industrial Congress, 57

industrialization, 27

industry regulation, 54

infantile paralysis. *See* polio

Infantile Paralysis Commission, 120

influenza, 30, 32; and mortality, 30, 31 (tab. 1), 32, 34 (tab. 2), 37, 40–41n19; twentieth-century epidemics of, 37, 202–203

inoculation. *See* vaccination

inspection, 16, 36, 156, 166, 183; and cholera, 160, 163; of meat and milk, 9, 14, 36, 157

intemperance, 51

Irish immigrants, 51, 67, 71

isolation. *See* quarantine

Italian immigrants, 165; and health care, 74, 86n35, 87n38; polio associated with, 26, 66, 71–74, 76, 116–117

Jacobi, Dr. Abraham, 158, 160, 179, 187n28, 193–194n129

Jacobson, Henning, 108–109

Jacobson v. *Massachusetts*, 108–109

Jacobus, Dr. Arthur M., 193n126

Janeway, Dr. Edward G., 160, 193n117

JCRS. *See* Jewish Consumptive Relief Society

Jenkins, Dr. William, 161

Jewish Consumptive Relief Society (JCRS), 80, 81–82

Jewish Hospital Association of Denver, 79

Jewish immigrants, 2, 87n40; polio associated with, 73, 116, 117; tensions between German and Eastern European, 79, 81, 82, 89n58, 90n75; tuberculosis associated with, 26, 74–75, 76–77, 78

Johns Hopkins Medical School, 157, 187n20
Johnson, Sterling, 141
Johnson administration, 206
Joseph, Stephen, 139–140, 141, 142, 143, 144

Kapp, Friedrich, 67
Kennedy, Edward, 145
Kenny, Elizabeth, 122–123
Kinyoun, Dr. Joseph, 69, 185n3
Klebs, Edwin, 165
Knopf, S. A., 13
Koch, Edward, 138, 140, 141, 142
Koch, Robert, 69, 155, 188n45, 195n147; bacteriologists studying under, 157, 186n15; and a cure for tuberculosis, 12, 176; tuberculosis bacillus discovered by, 11–12, 13, 75–76, 155, 156, 157, 175
Koprowski, Hilary, 126
Kortright, Dr. James, 173
Kramer, Larry, 134–135
Kraut, Alan M., 26, 84

labor market: and the eight-hour law, 59, 61; and housing, 42, 46–47, 54, 55–56, 58–59
labor movement, 51, 57, 60, 61
La Guardia, Fiorello, 184, 198, 199, 200, 205, 206
La Guerre, Herve, 65
Lambert, Alexander, 171
Lavinder, C. H., 72
law, 26, 43–44, 45–46, 47, 54, 55, 59, 62–63n8
Leavitt, Judith Walzer, 93, 188–189n51
Le Bar, Mr. and Mrs. Eugene, 95–96, 97, 102
Lederle, Ernst J., 180–181, 183
Lederle Antitoxin Laboratories, 181
Liebenau, Jonathan, 181
life expectancy, 28, 32, 40n18, 184
Lindsay administration, 207
Lister, Sir Joseph, 12
Loeffler, Friedrich, 165, 167
Longmuir, Mrs. A. O., 84n7

Loomis, Alfred, 157
Loomis, Henry P., 175–176
Low, Seth, 179, 180, 181, 194n135
Ludmerer, Kenneth M., 185n2, 186n14

McGrath, Diane, 138
McKeown, Thomas, 35, 36, 87–88n42
McLaughlin, Mary, 204
MacLean, Alistair, 127
McNeill, William, 131
malaria, and mortality, 34 (tab. 2), 40–41n19
Mallon, "Typhoid" Mary, 167, 189n59
Manhattan Company, 42
March of Dimes. See National Foundation for Infantile Paralysis
Mass, Dr. Lawrence, 134
Massachusetts, 155, 183
Maternity Center Association, 110
Mayo-Smith, Richmond, 72
measles, and mortality, 32, 34 (tab. 2), 40–41n19
meat inspection. See under inspection
medical profession, 44, 58, 156; and the health depatment, 16, 159, 164, 166–167, 171, 172, 173, 175, 176–179, 180, 182–183, 184, 188n40, 189–190n60, 193n126, 193–194n129, 195n151; individual predisposition to disease believed by, 9–11; interest groups within, 164, 199–200; medical histories taken by, 11–12
Medical Record, 162, 177
meningitis, 40n13; and mortality, 30, 31 (tab. 1), 32, 34 (tab. 2), 40–41n19
Metropolitan Board of Health, 33, 34, 59, 103, 105, 106, 107, 153
Metropolitan Health Act of 1866, 107
Milbank Memorial Fund, 196n154, 199
milk inspection. See under inspection
Mitchel, John P., 71
model tenement movement, 56
Modern Rise of Population, The (McKeown), 87–88n42
Monaghan, Frank, 110
Montefiore Echo, 79, 89n56

Montefiore Home for Chronic Invalids, 78–79
Morning Courier and Enquirer, 55
mortality rates, 3, 25, 39n5, 51, 52, 53, 55, 60 (*see also under specific diseases*); age patterns of, 33, 34 (tab. 2), 40n18, 56; changing pattern of, 14–15, 27–28, 29 (fig.1), 31 (tab. 1), 32–33, 34 (tab. 2), 35, 36–37, 39–40n12; and class differences, 42, 56; and endemic disease, 32, 38; and epidemics (*see* epidemics: and mortality); and immigrants, 9, 42, 53–54, 56, 66–67; in New York City, 29 (fig. 1), 30, 31 (tab. 1), 33, 39–40n12, 42, 183; in rural areas, 27–28; in urban areas, 27, 28, 35
Mott, Valentine, 4
Murphy, Charles F., 179–180, 194n133
Murphy, Michael, 179
Myers, Woodrow, 142–143

National Foundation for Infantile Paralysis, 119, 121–123, 124, 125, 126, 127–128
National Institutes of Health, 125
National Jewish Hospital for Consumptives, 79–80, 81–82, 90n75
National Tuberculosis Association, 121
nativism, 2, 26. *See also* immigrants: blamed for epidemics
New York Academy of Medicine, 158, 160, 161, 170, 178, 187n29, 193n117
New York Citizens' Association, 3, 15–16
New York City, 18, 155; bacteriology lab in, 155–156, 185n3; as center for polio epidemics, 115, 128n2; demographic and physical transformation of, in nineteenth century, 2, 202; as epicenter of AIDS epidemic, 131, 133; in the nineteenth century, 2–14; selective memory applied to history of, 1–2, 19n1
New York City Board of Education, 107, 113n24

New York City Board of Health. *See* Metropolitan Board of Health
New York City Department of Hospitals, 199
New York City Health Department, 18, 198; and AIDS, 135–136, 137, 138, 139–140, 142; bacteriology lab, 156, 157, 161, 162, 163, 164, 170–171, 177–182, 184, 191n80; budget and funding for, 14, 182, 183, 184; Bureaus of, 138, 156; and cholera, 30, 158, 160, 161, 162, 182, 203; creation of, 8, 203; decline of, 208n1, 208n2; demographic changes ignored by, 202; and diphtheria, 166–167, 168–169, 169, 170–171, 173–175, 189–190n60, 190n61, 190n75, 190–191n78; and environmental hazards, 8, 14–16; Medical Advisory Board of, 158–159, 163, 190n75; and the medical profession (*see* medical profession: and the health department); and pharmaceutical manufacturers, 180–181; and polio, 73, 116–117; political scandal in, 158–160, 163, 182, 187n28; and the politics of accretion, 205; and the politics of crisis, 210n16; and the politics of reform, 206; reputation of, 8, 181, 182–184, 195n147; and smallpox, 95, 96, 97, 99, 102, 109, 110, 112n3, 112n4; and Tammany Hall, 158–160, 163, 172, 179, 180, 194n131; tenement residents as "clinical material" for, 163–164, 171–172, 173, 188–189n51; and tuberculosis, 155, 157, 177, 193n117, 193n126, 193–194n129, 194n141, 195n147, 195n151; and typhoid fever, 156, 164; women hired by, 171
New York Civil Liberties Union, 137
New York County Medical Society, 177, 178
New York Diet Kitchen Association, 110
New York Herald, and diphtheria antitoxin, 169–170, 172, 190–191n78
New York Medical Journal, 159–169, 187n28

New York State Health Department, 140, 144

New York Times, 65, 110, 159; and the diphtheria antitoxin, 168, 173, 191–192n99, 193n125

New Zealand, 27, 39n5

Nobel Prize, 122, 127

Norwegian immigrants, 84n7

Novy, Frederick, 186n15

Oberwager, Dr. John, 120

O'Dwyer, William, 99, 111, 112n3

"1,112 and Counting" (Kramer), 134–135

Page, Catherine Sefton, 117

Page, Walter Hines, 117

Panic: of 1837, 53; of 1873, 60

Park, William Hallock, 161, 184, 196n154; and the antitoxin for diphtheria, 168, 169, 170, 173–174, 175, 190n75; and bacteriological research on diphtheria, 165–166, 167; as manager of the bacteriology lab, 117–118, 171, 181–182, 184

Parker, Willard, 4

Pasteur, Louis, 11, 12, 158

Pasteur Institute, 117

Pearl, Bertha, 79

PHANYC. *See* Public Health Association of New York City

pharmaceutical industry, 180–181, 184, 195n151

Philadelphia, 3, 183, 205; cholera in, 39n11, 52; yellow fever in, 27, 28

Philip, John R., 210n16

PHS. *See* United States Public Health Service

phthisis. *See* tuberculosis

physicians. *See* medical profession

plague, 69

Plagues and People (McNeill), 131

pneumonia, 15; mortality from, 32, 33, 34 (tab. 2)

polio, 18; causes of, 72, 93–94, 118, 120, 123; controlled after World War II, 14, 207, 210n16; as disease of cleanliness, 94, 122; epidemic of 1916, 37, 70, 115, 117–118, 119; epidemics of, 70–71, 73, 119, 120, 122, 123–124, 203; fund-raising for, 119, 120–121; as immigrant dirt disease, 26, 66, 71–74, 76, 84n7, 86n31, 115, 116–117, 118, 119, 122, 128; mortality rate of, 37, 71, 115, 119, 123; perceptions of victims of, 115, 124, 127, 128; preventive measures against, 37, 93, 94, 116–117, 119–120, 123; scientific research into, 115–116, 121–128; serum developed for, 117, 120; treatment for, 117, 122

Polio Surveillance Unit, 126

Polish immigrants, 73

"Politics in the Health Department," 159

population growth, 18; and housing, 51–52; and mortality, 27, 35, 42

poverty and the poor, 1, 26, 51; and AIDS, 16, 140, 147; disease associated with, 2, 13, 16, 25, 32, 44, 48, 51, 117, 153; and public health services, 198, 199, 200–202, 206, 207

Practitioners Society of New York, 190n61

Providence, Rhode Island, 155, 185n3, 189n59

Prudden, Dr. Theopil Mitchell, 157, 163; and the antitoxin for diphtheria, 169, 170, 190n75; and cholera, 160, 161, 162; and the laboratory at Columbia College, 157, 165; resignation from health department of, 158, 159, 187n28; and tuberculosis control, 175–176, 177, 178–179, 193n117, 193–194n129

public health, 93, 155, 196n152 (*see also* health); decline or growth in activities of, 197, 208n1, 208n2; definition of, 153–154, 197–198; and epidemics, 202–203, 207; focus of program for, 9, 14, 16, 156, 202; and funding, 184, 205, 207; and interest groups, 199–200, 208; and politics, 94, 184, 196n155, 197, 198–204, 205–208,

208–209n3, 210n16; and voluntary
agencies, 199, 209n6
Public Health Association of New York
City (PHANYC), 154
Pulmonary Tuberculosis (Fishberg), 76

quarantine, 9, 29, 36, 45, 93, 193n126;
and AIDS, 138, 142; and cholera, 28,
153, 158, 160–161, 162; and diphtheria, 167–168, 189–190n60; and
immigration, 66, 68, 69; and polio, 72,
73, 87n38, 116; and smallpox, 93,
103, 108; and tuberculosis, 78; and
yellow fever, 153

rabies, 11, 158
racism, 1, 2, 65
Radical Republicans, 59
Rangel, Charles, 141
Raske, Kenneth, 145
Reagan, Ronald, 140
Right-to-Life Party, 137
Riis, Jacob, 163–164
Riley, Thomas J., 73
Rivers, Dr. Tom, 99, 111, 112n4
Robbins, Frederick, 122
Rockefeller Foundation, 205
Rockefeller Institute for Medical Re-
search, 73, 84n7, 99, 115–116, 122,
184
Roosevelt, Eleanor, 118
Roosevelt, Franklin Delano, 93, 118–
119, 120, 121, 125, 128
Roosevelt, Robert, 3–4
Rosenau, M. J., 108
Rosenberg, Charles, 9, 16, 18, 50, 131,
171
Ross, E. A., 75
Ryan White Act, 146

Sabin, Albert, 115, 124–125, 126–127
Salk, Jonas, 115, 124–127, 128
San Francisco, California, 135, 136
Sanitary Condition of the City, 3–7, 8,
14

*Sanitary Conditions of [New York's] La-
boring Population* (Griscom), 4, 54
sanitation, 3, 4, 6–7, 9, 15, 35, 37, 53,
71, 156
Satan Bug, The (MacLean), 127
scarlet fever, 203; and mortality, 34 (tab.
2), 35, 40–41n19
Schaeffer, Morris, 196n154
Scheele, Leonard, 126
Schiff, Jacob, 78
Seaman, Dr. Valentine, 44, 104
Sedgwick, William T., 185n3
Sencer, David, 135–136, 137, 139, 141,
142
sewers, 8, 9, 14, 36, 45, 52–53, 54
Sexton, John B., 179
Shlevin, Ida May, 66
Shrady, Dr. George, 159, 162
*Silent Travelers: Germs, Genes, and the
"Immigrant Menace"* (Kraut), 84
Silverman, Mervyn, 136
smallpox, 2, 7, 10, 14, 18, 32, 69, 188–
189n51, 193–194n129; and the bacteriology lab of the health department,
156; case-tracing of, 99, 102, 111; and
civil liberties, 93, 107; epidemic of
1947 of, 95–102, 106, 107, 111; history of, in New York City, 102–111,
114n25; and mortality, 15, 27, 30, 31
(tab. 1), 32, 33, 34 (tab. 2), 35, 40–
41n19, 93, 102–103, 111; and public
compliance with vaccination campaign, 102, 103; symptoms of, 95, 103
Smallpox Hospital, 107, 108, 114n25
Smith, Dr. Stephen, 4, 158–159, 160,
187n28
Social Security, 198, 205, 206
Society of Medical Jurisprudence and
State Medicine, 105
Sontag, Susan, 83
Special Investigation of Infantile Paral-
ysis, 73
Specter, Michael, 88n51
Spivak, Dr. Charles, 80–81
State Hospital Review and Planning
Council, 201
Stoddard, Lothrop, 194n135

Straus, Nathan, 179, 193n125
street cleaning, 8, 36, 45, 54, 153, 156, 160, 162
Strong, William, 172
Substance Abuse Services, 135
swine flue, 135
syphilis, 16, 141; transferred through smallpox vaccination, 105, 106

Tammany Hall, 58, 158–160, 163, 168, 172, 179, 180, 181, 194n131
Tatum, Wilbert, 141
Taylor, Graham, 13, 14
Teaford, John, 46
Thatcher, John S., 190n75
Thoms, William, 6
Tobey, James, 109
Tolle, Dr. Dorothea M., 95, 96
Toner, Dr. J. M., 106–107
trachoma, 26, 69–70
Tracy, Roger, 11
Trudeau, Edward L., 77, 179
Truman, Harry S., 99
tuberculin, 176
tuberculosis, 1, 17, 28, 30, 70, 76, 94, 209n6; and age-standardized mortality, 33, 34 (tab. 2), 38, 75; and AIDS, 128, 142, 147; antitoxin for, 178–179, 180–181, 193n125; bacillus discovered for (see Koch, Robert: tuberculosis bacillus discovered by); compulsory reporting of, 155, 177–178, 193n117, 193–194n129, 203; decline of, 87–88n42; diagnosis of, 10, 11, 12, 70, 176–177; and employment, 10, 11, 12, 13–14; and immigrants, 26, 54, 70, 74–75, 76–77, 78, 89n56; and mortality, 3, 10, 15, 25, 29 (fig. 1), 32, 33, 35, 38, 75–76, 87–88n42, 175, 176, 177, 203; prevention program for, 13, 157, 175–176; recent cases of, 17, 78, 88n51, 147; and the sanitarium, 77–82, 87–88n42; and socioeconomic class, 10, 13, 16, 75, 77, 87n41, 177; treatment of, 10, 77, 78, 183

typhoid fever, 2, 10, 17, 32, 37, 156, 164, 184; mortality rates of, 15, 27, 30, 31 (tab. 1), 32, 34 (tab. 2), 40–41n19
"Typhoid" Mary Mallon, 167, 189n59
typhus, 7, 17, 32, 37, 40n13, 67, 69, 193–194n129; and mortality, 27, 30, 31 (tab. 1), 32, 40–41n19

United Hebrew Charities, 76, 79
United Hospital Fund, 146
United States, 75, 76, 155, 185n2; changes in mortality rates in, 27, 39n5
United States Congress, 68, 146, 206
United States Constitution, 109
United States House of Representatives, 146
United States Public Health Service (PHS), 69, 99, 102
United States Senate, 146
United States Supreme Court, 108–109

vaccination, 9, 15, 16, 135; compulsory, 96, 107, 108–109; and diphtheria (see diphtheria: antitoxin for); and personal rights and civil liberties, 93, 106, 108–109; and polio, 94, 115, 122, 124–127, 203; and school attendance, 107–108, 109, 113n24; and smallpox, 93, 95, 97–98, 99, 100 (fig. 7), 101 (fig. 8), 102, 103–106, 110, 112n3, 113n16, 184, 185, 191n91; and state power, 106, 107, 108, 109, 110, 111
Valentine, Bertha, 173
Van Wyck, Robert, 179
variolation. See vaccination
Vaughan, Victor C., 185n3, 186n15
venereal disease, 161, 203. See also syphilis
virology, 121–122, 124
Vladeck, Bruce, 146–147

Wagner, Robert, 204
Walker, Jimmy, 119
Walker, Wyatt, 141
Ward, Benjamin, 141
Warm Springs Foundation, 119, 121

water supplies, 8, 9, 14, 42, 45, 48, 52, 54, 205; and cholera, 160, 161, 162; and landords, 52–53; and mortality rates, 35, 36

Weaver, Harry, 123, 124, 125

Webster, Dr. Noah, 44

Weinstein, Israel, 97, 99, 111, 112n3, 112n4

Welch, William Henry, 157, 161, 174, 186n14, 187n20, 191–192n99

Weller, Thomas, 122

whooping cough, 32, 34 (tab. 2)

Willard Parker Hospital, 95, 96, 97, 98, 102, 187n29

Williams, Anna W., 171

Wilson, Charles, 158, 159, 160, 161, 162, 172, 177, 187n28, 188n33

Wilson, Leonard G., 87–88n42

Winchell, Walter, 125

Winslow, C.-E. A., 170

Winters, Dr. Joseph, 174, 175, 178

Workman's Circle of New York, 80

World Health Organization, 126

World War II, 76, 111, 205

Wynne, Dr. Shirley, 119, 120

Yates, Cotton, 85n31

yellow fever, 17, 28, 30, 32, 37, 48–49, 75; immigrants inspected for, 2, 69; medical investigations of, 44, 45; and mortality rates, 27, 30, 31 (tab. 1), 40–41n19; and poverty, 2, 7, 25, 44; responses to, 28, 48, 153

Young, William Harvey, 115

Zederbaum, Dr. Adolph, 82

zymotic diseases, 39n8